# *Smart Eats,*
# *Smart Supplements,*
# *and*
# *Smart Exercise*

# *Smart Eats,*

# *Smart Supplements,*

# *and*

# *Smart Exercise*

DUSTY R. GREEN, B.S., M.ED.

*Published by Natural Health Solutions*

Cover photography by David "Smiley" Irvin
Book design, cover, and layout by Stacy Hagstrom
Editor: Joe Norton, Ph.D.
Copy editors: Suzanne Ancy, Belia Freedman, and Rob Stuart, Ph.D.

Published by Natural Health Solutions, P.O. Box 9407 Fort Worth, Texas 76147

To order the book contact Natural Health Solutions above or via the internet at: http://www.spindle.net/dusty or call local: 817-868-0220 or 1-800-484-9479, code 1825.

Library of Congress Catalog Card Number: 96-092793
ISBN: 0-9655254-0-6

Green, Dusty, 1952-
        Smart Eats, Smart Supplements, and Smart Exercise.

Authors first edition--2,500 copies

**Disclaimer**
*This book was written to provide you with information.*
*Before beginning this or any other nutritional/medical regimen, consult a competent nutritional/medical professional. This book is not intended to replace medical advice. Any medical questions should be addressed to your physician.*
*I am a research scientist who is presenting information based on a compilation of scientific literature combined with successes my clients, friends, family, and I have experienced. Do not take the contents of this book as "gospel." I encourage you to check out other sources on these subjects to help you fully understand what your body is all about. It is totally and entirely your choice and responsibility if you decide to try anything mentioned in this book.*

I dedicate this book to my family, friends, and clients who have helped support me monetarily, mentally, and otherwise. I am very blessed to be surrounded by such wonderful people. This three year project has been very rewarding with all of you standing by my side as the "Doubting Thomases" express their messages. I am truly grateful to all of you for having the faith and confidence to believe in me. To attempt to name all of you would be unfair because I may inadvertantly leave someone out. Each of you know how bound in gratitude I am.

No one can do it like Mom who has always been there for me no matter what. She has always given me her complete support without doubt or question. Comments such as "Do you need this?....Do you have that?....How many of these do I take?"....without hesitation and total trust. She has unquestionably given me the independence and freedom to think and express my views without restraint.

# CONTENTS

## SECTION II

## SECTION III

# INTRODUCTION

Discovery and recovery.

They are what this book is all about.

The process began about 25 years ago when I graduated from high school in Azle, Texas. Shortly thereafter, in the Spring of 1972, The University of North Texas (UNT) opened its doors to me to pursue a bachelor's degree in Physical Education. University officials have since changed the name of that degree to Kinesiology, which is basically the study of human movement. In 1976, after completing the requirements for the degree, I jumped right into graduate school at UNT, being awarded a teaching fellowship at the same time. I was elated to think that a 23 year old from "Small Town, USA," would be teaching college level classes, much less getting any kind of degree. The small town environment generally does not encourage the pursuit of college degrees. My mom and I were the first to get college degrees in our family. She received her Bachelor and Master of Elementary Education from Texas Women's University in 1977 and 1982 respectively. I received my Masters of Education in 1978.

I moved from Denton, Texas, (UNT) to Houston, Texas, to take a job teaching in public school. I taught biology and physical education and coached football, basketball, and track for three years. It was not a pleasant experience. I had all this wonderful knowledge to impart and realized I was hired to be a disciplinarian for "peanuts." It really bummed me out.

For the next six years the real estate business was my calling. I moved back to the Dallas-Fort Worth area and invested in and built homes. When the bottom dropped out of the industry in 1986-1987, I went back to teaching, this time on the college level. It was no more "Mr. Disciplinarian" because most of the students actually appreciated the knowledge. They motivated me to learn more because of their quest for knowledge. I taught a lecture class that proved to be a natural lead-in for what I was about to discover. In the class, the curriculum covered smart exercise techniques and briefly touched on nutrition. I could not answer the students' nutrition questions as I wanted because I knew nothing about it. We were not taught anything about nutrition in college; and as I later learned, medical schools do not teach doctors about it; hence my serious research began. Because I only taught a few classes, I had time to do research, interpret studies, write about my findings, and establish my health counseling business. The findings have had a monumental effect on my own health and the health of my clients.

I was 35 years of age when I began teaching college level courses and was aging fast. Arthritis, bunions, hemorrhoids, tendinitis, frequent colds and flu, signs of skin cancer, and low energy levels plagued me, even though I jogged, played racquetball, cycled, played golf (walking mostly), lifted weights, and occasionally played volleyball, basketball, and tennis. I lived with the pain as if it were the "natural aging process."

And the medical profession was no help.

Their typical response was to "take ibuprofen, let me give you *this* or *that* prescription, or let me cut on you." Or "maybe in six months, your body will have enough time to heal itself, but in the meantime take painkillers." Pain killers mask the pain but do not heal the problem. I have never been "cut on" and do not want to be. Furthermore, I was not crazy about prescription drugs because of the harmful side effects and expense. I knew there had to be a better way....and there is.

At the age of 44, I have now found the solutions to the ailments mentioned above and many others that beset many of my clients. The solutions are simple. They are *Smart Eats, Smart Supplements, and Smart Exercise*. All three are necessary to achieve the goal of living and feeling better and reversing or preventing viral infections and disease. Smart eats alone help, but you will run the risk of nutritional deficiencies which show up as viral infections and disease. Smart supplements alone help, but you will not be able to lose or control body fat effectively. Smart exercise alone will put you only into the same shape that I used to be....not an enviable level. I know many overfat regular exercisers who are in bad health.

My method of research involves (1) a thorough examination of the literature that pertains to the subject; (2) personally trying the product or technique first and recommending it if I feel that it can be of benefit to my clients; and (3) reporting successes that clients have had that may not have pertained to me. I report only on those clients whom I am in contact with regularly.

Benefits of getting into this three-pronged program are that you will:

1. feel great all the time;
2. develop a stronger immune system;
3. get rid of that pesky disease or condition that you currently have;
4. lower your probability of getting a virus or disease;
5. spend less time and money at the doctor or hospital;
6. spend less or no money on prescriptions;
7. spend less money and time on foods and food preparation;
8. lose body fat the right-healthy-smart way without starvation;
9. actually enjoy the taste and variety of the foods you will be eating;
10. heal much faster if injured;
11. be more mentally sharp;
12. be able to perform better physically;
13. recover from exercise much faster;
14. get hooked on exercise; *and*
15. savor the sexual experience (or maybe start again).

—Dusty R. Green, BS., M.ED.
Fort Worth, Texas
January, 1997

## THE GREATEST GAME IN THE WORLD

The games we enjoy most are the ones that are fun and challenging. View this process (the whole book) as a game that has been created for you—*a game in which you learn the rules that make you a winner for the rest of your life.* You will discover inner positive characteristics about yourself not previously known to you. Each day will be a stepping stone for a new and refreshing challenge awaiting you. To get the full benefit of the book, practice what is suggested as you read it. If you encounter an area you do not fully comprehend either; read it again; cross-reference other authorities mentioned in this book; or seek other information on the subject in libraries and/or bookstores.

# Section I

*Smart Eats*

# CHAPTER 1

## SMART EATS

Eating smart is the first step toward good health. Eating smart may mean you will have to make a slight change in your eating habits, but for most of us that will be a positive change. You will be surprised at just how quick, cheap and easy it is to eat five meals a day. Dusty's Lowfat Fare, below is a prototype for you to follow. Adjust the calorie numbers according to your weight, which you will find on page 42. As your weight changes (if that is your desire), your numbers will change accordingly.

## DUSTY'S LOWFAT FARE

**Breakfast**- All Bran, Fiber One, or any other high fiber cereal mixed with your favorite cereal. Use 1/2 percent or skim milk. This combination will be 300-400 calories with about 3-4 percent of your calories from fat. If you do not like cereal, most fruits and vegetables are high in fiber. See page 15 for more information on fiber.

**2nd meal, 3 hours later**- 1 sports bar with water;  220-300 calories;  8-13 percent of calories from fat.

**3rd meal, 3 hours later**- Healthy Choice chicken fajitas with water;  200 calories;  14 percent of calories from fat.

**4th meal, 3 hours later**- Tuna sandwich on wheat mixed with no fat dressing and relish;  one banana and water;  300 calories;  5 percent of calories from fat.

**5th meal, 3 hours later**- Medium baked potato with no fat sour cream, dressing, or salsa, and no fat cheese with 8 ounces of skim milk:  400 calories; 6 percent of calories from fat.

Always include fruits and/or vegetables in at least two of the five meals. They contain large amounts of fiber and potassium. More on that later. "Pig out" on the weekends or any 2 days of the week eating high fat foods if you like, but stay within the range of calories consistent with your body size (see page 42) to lose or maintain body fat.

# I DON'T HAVE TIME TO EAT THAT OFTEN!

Many people think they do not have time to eat five times a day. The above meals and the ones on page 32 are quick and easy to prepare. Eating them takes only 10 to 15 minutes.  Most people have several breaks during the day that can accommodate this eating style and most of these meals can be carried in your pocket, purse, or sports bag. If you eat breakfast and the fifth meal at home, then you have only three meals to eat at work or school.

# CHAPTER 2

## WHY SO MANY MEALS?

Those of you who eat only one, two or three meals per day experience the "blood sugar roller coaster." During and immediately following the big meal, you feel "up." Then one to three hours later you are "down" and ready for a nap. Most of us have been raised to believe that three heavy square meals per day is the way to do it. That pattern sets us up for hypoglycemia, diabetes, or just the blahs. Eating smaller meals about three hours apart helps to keep blood sugar levels consistently up and lowers stomach volume, allowing the stomach to feel full on smaller amounts of food. Those who eat one and/or two meals per day particularly send the body a message that it is being starved, and it tends to hold on to as much body fat as possible. If you are a one or two mealer, you will continue to have a hard time getting rid of fat. Three meals per day is not quite as bad, but you still experience the biological pitfalls of the rise and fall in blood sugar and erratic release of insulin.

Consider our ancestors who used to hunt for and/or grow their own food. Most of them ate frequently and expended a lot of energy hunting and dragging it around. When they did not find it for a day or so (an unintentional fast), their bodies had to be able to survive. The survival mechanism is the process that the body utilizes by holding on to body fat. That

5

same process is a part of our biological make-up today. The problem is that most of us "fast" every day of the week by only consuming one to three meals per day in our traditional style. As a result, most of us carry dangerously high amounts of stored body fat.

## Insulin-Like Growth Factor (IGF)

Another big boost for eating every three hours has to do with the release of insulin-like-growth factor (IGF) from the liver. This is the compound that travels to muscle cells and encourages muscular growth. IGF acts directly on muscle by putting amino acids into muscle cells. In order for IGF to do its job, there has to be a consistent and sufficient supply of insulin, which is released by the pancreas. Consuming five meals per day establishes a consistent and sufficient supply of insulin from the pancreas. Since insulin helps to maintain the level of sugar in the blood, a steady stream of insulin from the pancreas and IGF from the liver is crucial for muscle growth. The rise and fall of insulin on a one, two, or three meal per day disrupt the anabolic (muscle growth) drive—as on your "pig out" days. That is why you want to limit those days to only two.

## Growth Hormone Release...
## The True Fountain of Youth?

I have often been asked "Isn't it bad to eat in the evening hours?" It is true that when you go to sleep your pituitary gland releases growth hormone. Growth hormone release helps the body use fat for fuel, building muscle, enhancing the power of the immune system, expediting the healing process, and increasing skin thickness to that of our teen years. About the age of 30, the release declines dramatically. Exercising large muscle groups (legs and buttocks) aerobically and anaerobically (see Section III) encourages growth hormone release. These traits are characteristic of us in our teen years. Food in the stomach at exercise and bedtime reduces the effectiveness of the pituitary in releasing growth hormone. Many studies and continuing research shows that we can turn the production back to our teen years by eating, supplementing, and exercising smart. If you are consuming only 200-500 calories (depending on your weight) at or around 9 p.m., your stomach has emptied by 11 o'clock to midnight. On the traditional 800-1,500 calories evening meal, your stomach will empty much later thus interfering with the nighttime function of the pituitary.

**The bottom line is calories in and calories out!** If you have a caloric deficit at the end of the week, then you have lost some body fat. If it happens to be a 3,500 caloric deficit, then you have lost a pound.

8

# CHAPTER 3

## PERCENTAGE OF CALORIES FROM FAT

Following the eating plan in Chapter 1 will put your percentage of calories from fat in the 10-20 percent range. The other percentages of food content will vary between 60-68 percent of the calories from carbohydrates and 15-25 percent of the calories from protein (keep protein consumption at 15 percent or below if you are not currently involved in an exercise program....see page 105 on protein consumption). These percentages include the two days of "piggin' out." Most restaurants cuisine constitutes 35-45 percent of the calories from fat. If you do not eat out that often, then you may want to keep some high fat foods at home to satisfy that "high fat fix" that some of us so desperately desire on our two "piggin' out" days. If you are like most of us, dining at our favorite restaurant once or twice per week is our reward for that week. You are likely to lose weight faster if the "piggin' out" part of the plan is omitted; however, if you try to go "cold turkey" on this low fat fare, you may burn yourself out and become part of the well known statistic: "95 percent of those who diet, end up gaining back more weight than they originally started with." This book is not promoting a "diet" as such—it is providing an eating plan that you can follow for the rest of your life.

# Processed Junk

Most of the foods in my eating plan are packaged and processed. These packaged and processed foods have had the life sucked right out of them and their nutritional values are nil. Even though the majority of these foods are devoid of valuable vitamins, minerals, amino acids, and enzymes, they are full of complex and simple carbohydrates that become our body's main fuel source. Complex and simple carbohydrates are an undeniable necessity. There are better foods (made from scratch and foods purchased from whole food markets) available; yet obtaining or preparing them can be difficult or time consuming. If you have the resources and the time, then I strongly encourage you to prepare your foods from "scratch" or consume foods purchased from whole food markets.

Those who insist junk food has no nutritional value or are "empty calories" do not always realize that *most* of our food sources have negligible nutritional values. Whole foods and meals made from scratch fare a little better, but certainly do not solve our nutritional deficiencies. A lack of vitamins, minerals, amino acids, and enzymes in our daily diet are precisely why Section II, Smart Supplements is such an integral part of this program.

For those of you who like to prepare from scratch, there are many good low-fat recipe books at your local bookstore. Most of them give calorie information, but you may have to figure the percentage of calories from fat on your own. Some recipes in books are not very low in fat. If a recipe has more than 20 percent of the calories from fat, discard it unless you can bring your average down during the day or week with other low fat foods. Apple sauce and prune puree are great substitutes in recipes that call for butter and oils as ingredients. You cannot tell the difference in taste, and are replacing near 100 percent of the calories from fat with carbohydrates high in fiber.

# Figuring Percentage of Calories From Fat

*All of anything is 100 percent.*
A tablespoon of butter and/or most dressings and oils is about **100** calories.
It is all fat! 100 percent!

*Three fourths of anything is 75 percent.*
3 strips of bacon are about **100** calories.
About 75 of the 100 calories come from fat.

*Half of anything is 50 percent.*
A 1.23 oz. mint frosted brownie (Weight Watchers) is about **100** calories.
About 50 of the 100 calories come from fat.

*One third of anything is 33 percent.*
9 Barnum's Animal Crackers are about **100** calories.
About 33 of the 100 calories come from fat.

*One fourth of anything is 25 percent.*
1 oz. Baked Tostitos Cool Ranch Tortilla Chips is **120** calories.
30 of the 120 calories come from fat.

*One fifth of anything is 20 percent.*
1 Lunch Bucket Pasta and Chicken is **150** calories.
About 30 of the calories come from fat.

*One tenth of anything is 10 percent.*
A 6 ounce can of Star Kist chunk light tuna in spring water is **150** calories.
15 of the 150 calories come from fat.

*One twentieth of anything is 5 percent.*
About 1 cup of Kellogg's Frosted Mini-Wheats is **200** calories.
10 of the 200 calories come from fat.

....and so on.

Another way to ascertain the percentage of calories from fat is to divide the calories per serving (the big number) into the fat calories (the smaller number). For example; the Frosted Mini-Wheats above could be figured this way:

$$\textbf{calories per serving} = 200 \, \overline{)\, \textbf{10.00} = \textbf{fat calories}}^{\textbf{.05} = \textbf{percent of calories from fat}}$$

If you happen to be in the grocery store and do not have a calculator, you may find this next method easiest of all. Let us say the product has 200 calories per serving and 30 of those calories come from fat. Now start counting the number of 30s that will fit into 200 with your fingers. 30 (1 finger),.... 60 (2 fingers),.... 90 (3 fingers),.... 120 (4 fingers),.... 150 (5 fingers), and 180 (6 fingers). There are six 30's with a little to spare. Anything over 5 fingers or 1/5th is less than 20 percent. That is your goal. There is a "ton of food" out there that is less than 20 percent these days. Fill your cabinets and refrigerator with them.

Fast food restaurants have nutritional pamphlets that you can ask for that break down the fat, carbohydrate, and protein ratios—you should feel quite comfortable in asking to see a copy. Most other restaurants now are offering low fat plates.

# CHAPTER 4

## INTERPRETING FOOD LABELS

Now that you understand how to figure percentage of calories from fat, you are ready to shop smart. There are four main things to look for on the new nutrition facts label.

| | Nutrition Facts | |
|---|---|---|
| | **Serving Size 1 packet (28g)** | |
| | **Servings per container 2** | |
| | **Amount per serving** | |
| 1{ | Calories | 110 |
| 2{ | Calories from fat | 25 |
| | | **% Daily Value** |
| | Total Fat 2.5g | 4% |
| | Saturated Fat | 0% |
| | Cholesterol 0mg | 0% |
| 3{ | Sodium 160mg | 7% |
| | Potassium 110mg | 3% |
| | Total Carbohydrate 18g | 6% |
| 4{ | Dietary Fiber 3g | 12% |
| | Sugars 0g | |
| | Protein 3g | |

13

**1. Calories (per serving), 110.**

**2. Calories from fat, 25:** Count on your fingers how many separate 25's will fit into the 110 calories per serving. Four plus a little extra—not quite five giving you between 20 and 25 percent. Since you now have a cabinet full of foods below 20 percent, this food will be okay to consume. Average these newly acquired foods in your cabinets with this food, and you will find your total percentage of calories from fat below 20. The following list of foods on page 32-33 average about 15 percent of calories from fat. And as you can see, there are a couple that hover around the 30 percent mark.

**3. Sodium, 160 milligrams:** The Food and Nutrition Board (an arm of our government) says we should not exceed 2,400 milligrams per day. The widespread concern with sodium is good. We should be aware of the amounts we consume. Unfortunately, we are not being told the whole story. The Food and Drug Administration (FDA), another arm of our government, does not require potassium content to be put on labels. This label just happens to have it. What the FDA is not telling us is we should be consuming a potassium/sodium ratio of 2:1 in favor of potassium. Well-documented studies show populations with high-sodium, low-potassium intakes have a higher incidence of high blood pressure and stroke-related deaths, such as in the United States. Those same studies show that if sodium intake stays the same and potassium is increased to the 2:1 ratio as stated above, blood pressure and stroke-related deaths decline dramatically. See Section II, page 96 for more on sodium and potassium.

My concern therefore is that we should be consuming 3,000 milligrams of potassium to 1,500 milligrams of sodium...or 5,000 milligrams of potassium to 2,500 milligrams of sodium...or 6,000 milligrams of potassium to 3,000 milligrams of sodium per day and so on. If you find it difficult to cut back on sodium then increase your potassium intake and keep track of both your potassium and sodium intake. If you desire extra salt on your food, use salt substitute (potassium chloride) called *Nosalt*. Equally as smart, is to include *fresh fruits* and *vegetables* as two or three of your meals daily, providing high levels of both potassium and fiber.

**4. Dietary fiber, 3 grams:** It lowers cholesterol levels (a waxy-like substance that comes from animal related products and clogs our arteries). Fiber also lowers the incidence of diabetes, obesity, intestinal disorders, colon and rectum cancer, constipation, hemorrhoids, and heart disease. The typical American diet contains about 20 grams per day. *We need between 30 and 50 grams per day.* It makes us feel full by expanding in our stomachs and gathers carcinogenic (cancer causing) materials in the small and large intestines, which are then expelled in our newly made soft stools. As you begin to read labels regularly, you will see how easy it is to reach the 30-50 gram range....particularly if fresh fruits, vegetables, and grains become a regular part of your fare.

Since your number one objective is to search for 20 percent or less of the calories from fat, you will find that all the other things on the label are generally okay. If it is low in overall fat, it is low in saturated fats (mostly animal related--the kind that clogs arteries). If it is low in fat, it is high in carbohydrates (unless it is a meat product; then it is high in protein). If it is low in fat, it is low in cholesterol.

## WHAT ABOUT THE PERCENTAGE DAILY VALUE COLUMN?

Forget it! The numbers listed as "percentage daily value" are based on 2,000 calorie consumption. That is okay for the 180 pounder who gets no exercise and perhaps the 130 pounder who burns 700 calories per day over his or her BMR (see page 41) through exercise every day, and wants to maintain his or her weight. There are far too many variables that dictate whether or not we should be consuming 2,000 calories per day.

# CHAPTER 5

## LACTOSE INTOLERANT?....OR YOU JUST DON'T LIKE MILK.

For those of you who are lactose intolerant and are concerned about the amount of skim milk on the plan, make this adjustment: *eat fresh fruits and vegetables, which are high in both fiber and potassium.* Skim milk has no fiber but has about 400 milligrams of potassium per 8 ounces. You receive the benefit of both fiber and potassium from fresh, not processed, fruit. Unfortunately, canning and/or processing fruits and vegetables reverses the sodium/potassium ratio in favor of sodium. The ratio **before** canning and/or processing is about 7:1 in favor of potassium. After canning and processing, the ratio becomes about 3:1 in favor of sodium. For more information on potassium and sodium, see page 96 in Section II.

On the following page are some fresh foods that are high in potassium (Table 5-1).

**Table 5-1**

| Fresh Food | Portion | Potassium (mgs.) approximate |
|---|---|---|
| 1 Banana | medium | 600 |
| Tuna | 3.5 ozs. | 300 |
| Cantaloupe | half | 850 |
| Chicken | 3.5 ozs. | 300 |
| Skim Milk | 8 ozs. | 400 |
| Spinach | 3.5 ozs. | 800 |
| Potato | medium | 800 |
| Orange | medium | 350 |
| Carrots | 3.5 ozs. | 350 |
| Apple | medium | 350 |
| Celery | 3.5 ozs. | 150 |
| Avocado | medium | 750 |
| Salmon | 3.5 ozs. | 350 |
| Asparagus | 3.5 ozs. | 200 |

# CHAPTER 6

## GROCERY STORE FIELD TRIP

How can food manufacturers make these wonderful claims like "85 percent fat free," "90 percent fat free," etc.? In reality, these claims should send up the "The Red Flag." Upon examining the label, you will find that most of these claims really mean you are buying a product with 50 percent or more of the calories from fat per serving. They are basing their claims on total weight of the product. Take a look at this 100 gram (3.5 ounce) serving of turkey labeled "90 percent fat free."

**Table 6-1**

| Ingredient | Weight | Calories |
|------------|--------|----------|
| Water | 70 gms. | 0 |
| Fat | 10 gms. | 90 |
| Protein | 20 gms. | 80 |
| | | **170 total** |

Of the 170 total calories, 90 come from fat, which is a whopping *53 percent.*

## CARBOHYDRATE CRAZY

The two forms of carbohydrates you will be consuming on this plan are complex and simple. The *complex* variety includes fruits, grains, vegetables, and legumes. *Simple* carbohydrates come from sugars found in most candy bars, sport drinks, sodas, honey, cold cereals, breakfast bars, diet shakes, and the list goes on. Food manufacturers sometimes list the sugar ingredient as corn syrup, dextrose, sucrose, high fructose corn syrup, fruit juice concentrates, fructose, glucose, maltose, oligosaccharides, and monosaccharides. If any of these are listed at the beginning of the ingredients, the product has a large amount of sugar in it. Too much sugar can cause many health problems, especially if you are not a regular exerciser. Sugar is used as a quick burning fuel for the exercising muscles. Complex carbohydrates are longer lasting. Consider *simple* carbohydrates as the matches that start the fire, and *complex* as the logs that keep burning once the fire is lit. If you are concerned about the amount of sugar in some of the foods I recommend, do not eat packaged and processed foods, including cold cereals, SnackWells products, some Healthy Choice products, sodas, concentrated fruit juices, etc. The new labels tell you how many grams of simple and complex carbohydrates the product has per serving in this language:

**Total Carbohydrate = 26 grams (both simple and complex)**
**Dietary Fiber = 3 grams**
**Sugars = 10 grams**

The above carbohydrate, dietary fiber, and sugar amounts come from a packet of apples and cinnamon oatmeal. The label indicates there are 26 total grams of carbohydrates. It also states there are 10 grams of sugar, which are simple carbohydrates. If there are 10 grams of sugar, then there are 16 grams of complex carbohydrates: 26 grams minus 10 grams equals 16 grams. Three of the 16 grams of complex carbohydrates are in the form of dietary fiber.

We run into problems with sugar consumption in the typical western diet when we eat sugar coated cereals, pop tarts, breakfast bars, candy bars, cookies, cakes, ice cream, and sodas day to day. You have heard of drug overdoses? These foods cause a sugar overdose, particularly when no exercise is involved. The exercising body tolerates this amount of sugar much better than the non-exercising body.

# CHAPTER 7

## MY TYPICAL DAILY FARE

The following fare is a variation from the fare in Chapter 1. The two main differences are the calorie count and protein content. All other aspects of the two fares are similar in principle. I personally require more calories and protein content because I exercise. Calorie count (page 47) and protein content (page 105) are discussed more in detail later. *Dietary fiber and sugars are both part of the total carbohydrates.*

**9 a.m.**
*20 ozs. of reverse osmosis water (r.o.w. page 67) with supplements.*
*1 cup of black coffee.*
*1 cup of Cinnamon Life Cereal mixed with*
*1/4 cup sugar free All Bran and 8 ozs. of skim milk.*
Total fat = 4 grams x 9 calories per gram = 36 calories or about 10 per cent of the calories.
Total carbohydrates = 62 grams x 4 calories per gram = 248 calories or 71 percent of the calories.
Dietary fiber = 15 grams.
Sugars = 34 grams.

Total protein = 17 grams x 4 calories per gram = 68 calories or 19 percent of the calories.

*352 total calories.*

## Noon

*1-16oz. bag of Birds Eye broccoli, carrots, and water chestnuts with 2 pieces of Honey Wheat Berry bread and r.o.w.*
*One and one-half (1-1/2) serving of Designer Protein supplement (page 105)= 25 grams of protein.*

Total fat = 5 grams x 9 calories per gram = 45 calories or 10 percent of the calories.

Total carbohydrates = 68 grams x 4 calories per gram = 272 calories or 60 percent of the calories.

Dietary fiber = 19 grams.

Sugars = 17 grams.

Total protein = 35 grams x 4 calories per gram =140 calories or 31 percent of the calories.

*457 total calories.*

## 3 p.m.

*20 ozs. of r.o.w. with supplements.*
*One and one half (1-1/2) serving of Designer protein supplement = 25 grams of protein.*
*1 Life Extension cookie (page 33).*
*1 sports bars (No Holds Bar, Power Bar, or Edge Bar -page 33) with a 12 oz. Coke.*

Total fat = 7 grams x 9 calories per gram = 63 calories or 11 percent of the calories.

Total carbohydrates = 99 grams x 4 calories per gram = 396 calories or 66 percent of the calories.

Dietary fiber = 7 grams.

Sugars = 60 grams.

Total protein = 36 grams x 4 calories per gram = 144 calories or 24 per cent of the calories.

*603 total calories.*

**6 p.m.**

*20 ounces of r.o.w.*
*1 cup of Healthy Choice Cappuccino Chocolate Chunk ice cream*
*One and one half (1-1/2) serving of Designer Protein Supplement = 25*
*grams of protein.*

Total fat = 3 grams x 9 calories per gram = 27 calories or 9 percent of the
    calories.

Total carbohydrates = 37 grams x 4 calories per gram = 148 calories or
    49 percent of the calories.

Dietary fiber = 2 grams.

Sugars = 38 grams.

Total protein = 31 grams x 4 calories per gram = 124 calories or 41 per
    cent of the calories.

*299 total calories.*

**9 p.m.**

*6 ounces of r.o.w. with supplements.*
*1 Healthy Choice Chicken Enchiladas Suiza with a 12 ounce Coke.*

Total fat = 4 grams x 9 calories per gram = 36 calories or 9 percent of the
    calories.

Total carbohydrates = 82 grams x 4 calories per gram = 328 calories or
    80 percent of the calories.

Dietary fiber = 5 grams.

Sugars = 43 grams.

Total protein = 14 grams x 4 calories per gram = 56 calories or 13 percent
    of the calories.

*420 total calories.*

**11:30 p.m.**—goodnight!

**Total calories for the day = 2131.**

Total fat for the day = 23 grams x 9 calories per gram = 207 calories or
    about 10 percent of the calories from fat.

Total carbohydrates for the day = 348 grams x 4 calories per gram = 1,392
    calories or 66 percent of the calories from carbohydrates.

<u>Total grams of fiber</u> = 44.
<u>Total grams of sugars</u> = 192.
<u>Total protein for the day</u> = 133 grams x 4 calories per gram = 532 calories or 25 percent of the calories from protein.

This fare is perfect for me for losing body fat. It may be the perfect numbers for you too if you are about my weight, which is 160 lbs. If you are burning about 1,100 calories per day doing some type of aerobic activity (one and one-half hours of racquetball in this case) and your basal metabolic rate (BMR: the number of calories you burn while engaged in your normal sedentary everyday activities - see page 41 for more on BMR) is 1,700 calories per day, then (1,700+1,100) 2,800 calories per day is the total number of calories you are burning. Result: 2,800 calories burned minus 2,131 calories consumed equals a 669 calorie deficit. The 669 calorie deficit times five days equals 3,345 calories, equating to a loss of about a pound of body fat. Actually, a pound of body fat equates to approximately 3,500 calories.

# CHAPTER 8

## NOW LET'S "PIG OUT!"

Here comes the weekend or maybe it is a Wednesday and Saturday or any two day combination for you. It is mostly a Friday-Saturday or a Saturday-Sunday combination for me.

Let us consider the Friday-Saturday combination.

**Friday breakfast**

*20 ounces of r.o.w. with supplements.*
*1 Sports Bar = 230 calories.*
*1 Coke = 150 calories.*
*1 cup of black coffee = 0 calories.*

Percentage of calories from fat = 5 percent.

**2nd meal-noon**

*1 cantaloupe=200 calories.*

Percentage of calories from fat = 5 percent.

**3 p.m.**

*20 ounces of r.o.w. with supplements.*

*6 ozs. of tuna with fat free ranch and relish = 200 calories.*
Percentage of calories from fat = less than 5 percent.

**6.p.m.**
*2 light beers or 1 cocktail = 200 calories.*
Percentage of calories from fat = less than 5 percent.

**7.p.m.**
*1/2 of a medium Pizza Hut pepperoni/jalapeno pizza
and water = 1,150 calories.*
Percentage of calories from fat = 35 percent.

**Somewhere between 11:30 p.m. and 3 a.m.**
*6 ounces of r.o.w. with supplements.*

**Total calories for the day = 2,130.**
Percentage of calories from fat for the day = **20 percent.**

Sometime that afternoon I walked briskly (4 m.p.h. or so) for an hour. That equates to about 400 calories of expenditure plus the 1,700 calorie BMR totaling 2,100 calories. *That is 30 calories away from equaling the caloric intake for the day.*

**Saturday morning breakfast.**
*20 ounces of r.o.w. with supplements.*
*1 cup of Frosted Mini-Wheats with 1/4 cup of All Bran
and 8 ozs. of skim milk = 350 calories.*
Percentage of calories from fat = 5 percent.

**Noon.**
*Loaded Whataburger with cheese
with medium fries and a Coke = 1,200 calories.*
Percentage of calories from fat = 40 percent.

**3 p.m.**

*20 ounces of r.o.w. with supplements.*

**6 p.m.**

*Still full from the Whataburger.*

**9 p.m.**

*Supplements and 3 Snackwell's Devil's Food Cookies
with 8 ounces of skim milk = 250 calories.*
<u>Percentage of calories from fat</u> = less than 5 percent.

I consumed 1,800 calories and burned 1,700 as a result of my basal metabolic rate. I did not exercise and therefore, had a 100 calorie overage for the day. That 100 calorie overage is insignificant unless we start piling up a bunch of them. The percentage of calories from fat for Saturday was about 34 percent.

*The total percentage of calories for the week (all 7 days) was about 13 percent while losing about a pound of body fat!*

## ALL THAT SATURATED FAT!

You may ask, "What about all the saturated fat in the pizza and cheeseburger?" There is a lot of saturated fat in those foods. I recall a time when I used to eat that much saturated fat every day of the week. <u>Focus on weekly totals.</u> Thirteen percent for the week means your saturated fat intake for the week is very low. Part of that 13 percent is monounsaturated and polyunsaturated fats, which are much more friendly to your system than totally saturated fats. Too much of any kind of fat that is consumed and/or stored as body fat generates free radicals. Free radicals are the basis for accelerated aging and disease in all animals (more about free radicals in Section II). Humans and lab animals typically store more fat than humans and animals in the wild, which is why we need a plan such as the one that you are reading about.

# CHAPTER 9

## MORE SMART EATS

Below are some foods you may want to try, most all low in fat. Pay special attention to the fruits and vegetables because of the high potassium and fiber content. Most of the other foods, since they are processed, have at least a 1:1 ratio of potassium to sodium. Some have a 3:1 ratio in favor of sodium. Fresh fruits and vegetables generally have a 7:1 ratio in favor of potassium. Combine daily fruits and vegetables with daily low fat processed foods, and your heart and circulatory system will thank you very kindly.

All of these foods can be obtained at your grocery store, Sam's Wholesale, or sporting goods store (Power Bar, No Holds Bar, and Edge Bars). These bars among others can be bought in higher quantities for less money by calling their toll free numbers. Power Bar 1/800-444-5154, No Holds Bar 1/800-404-7974, and Edge Bar 1/800-659-7654. Life Extension Cookies can be purchased by calling 1/800-544-4440.

## Table 9-1.

| | Calories | Fat Calories | % Fat Calories |
|---|---|---|---|
| 1 Fresh Mango | 135 | 9 | 7 |
| Hungry Jack Microwave Pancakes w/lite syrup & fat free margarine | 320 | 36 | 11 |
| 1 El Charrito Burrito | 230 | 45 | 20 |
| 4 Delimex Beef Taquitos w/ salsa | 350 | 63 | 18 |
| 1-12 oz. bowl mixed fruit | 200 | 0 | 0 |
| 1-2oz. Angela Maries Marshmallow Munchie | 216 | 45 | 21 |
| 1 bag Microwave Bacon Curls w/fat free dressing | 250 | 36 | 14 |
| 1/2 bag Quaker Butter Popped Corn Cakes | 245 | 0 | 0 |
| 1 fresh cantaloupe | 200 | 0 | 0 |
| 1 oz. Stauffers Animal Crackers | 115 | 18 | 15 |
| Lunch Bucket Pasta and Chicken | 150 | 27 | 18 |
| Lunch Bucket Dumplings n Chicken | 110 | 18 | 16 |
| 1/2 fresh honeydew melon | 200 | 0 | 0 |
| 43 Crisp Baked Bugles | 90 | 18 | 20 |
| 2 servings oatmeal w/sugar and Butter Buds | 350 | 36 | 10 |
| All Healthy Choice Entrees | varies | varies | varies |
| 1-12 oz. bowl mixed vegetables | 150 | 0 | 0 |
| 1-12 oz. bowl of mixed salad w/ fat free dressing | 150 | 0 | 0 |
| 1/4 pound cheeseburger made w/extra extra lean beef, fat free cheese, fat free mayo., hot mustard, pickles, onion, lettuce, & tomato on wheat | 350 | 45 | 13 |
| 1 Double Decker Moon Pie | 250 | 54 | 22 |
| 1 banana | 100 | 0 | 0 |
| 1 Power Bar | 225 | 18 | 8 |
| 1 Edge Bar | 234 | 18 | 8 |
| 1 No Holds Bar | 330 | 60 | 18 |

| | Calories | Fat Calories | % Fat Calories |
|---|---|---|---|
| **1 serving Betty Crocker Tuna Helper, (using prune puree or apple sauce instead of butter)** | 220 | 36 | 16 |
| **1-12 oz. bowl fresh grapes** | 100 | 0 | 0 |
| **1 serving Mahatma Red Beans & Rice** | 190 | 5 | 3 |
| **1 cup (8 oz.) Blue Bell Light Ice Cream** | 220 | 45 | 20 |
| **1 cup Healthy Choice Ice Cream** | 240 | 40 | 17 |
| **1 serving Hains Honey Nut Mini Rice Cakes** | 60 | 0 | 0 |
| **1 medium baked potato w/ fat free ranch, fat free cheese, & chives** | 300 | 0 | 0 |
| **8 Nabisco Honey Maid Graham crackers** | 120 | 25 | 21 |
| **1 bag Betty Crocker Pop Secret Popcorn By Request Butter Flavor** | 260 | 50 | 19 |
| **1 Apple** | 80 | 0 | 0 |
| **1 Orange** | 70 | 0 | 0 |
| **1 oz. Baked Tostitos dipped in 1 oz. Healthy Choice Cheese Product w/salsa or Rotel** | 180 | 9 | 5 |
| **6 SnackWells Vanilla or Chocolate Creme cookies** | 300 | 54 | 18 |
| **Frozen fresh fruit smoothie (blend 1 banana, 5 strawberrys,and 1/2 cantaloupe)** | 250 | 0 | 0 |
| **1 Life Extension Cookie (Peanut Butter, Chocolate Chip, and Date Nut flavors)** | 120 | 45-50 | 38-42 |

The Life Extension Cookie shows a high percent of fat calories. A significant amount of those fat calories come from a fat called medium-chain triglycerides (MCTs), which change fat metabolism so that more fat is converted into energy. Unlike most common fatty acids (oils), MCTs metabolize quickly to provide energy (twice the caloric energy of carbohydrates). One cookie will give you the feeling of fullness as quick as one to two sports bars with fewer calories.

A book containing food calorie values such as *The Fat Counter* by Natow and Heslin will be a big help as you begin purchasing foods not mentioned in this book.

# CHAPTER 10

## LOW FAT MANIA

The benefits from eating low fat foods are many. Consuming 100 grams of fat totals 900 calories (9 calories per gram). Consuming 100 grams of carbohydrate or protein totals 400 calories (4 calories per gram). You will achieve the feeling of fullness (satiety) sooner by consuming 100 grams of carbohydrates as opposed to 100 grams of fat. That is 500 fewer calories! A single high carbohydrate meal triggers the release of cholycystokinin (CCK), which is a hormone that initiates the satiety center in the brain making you feel full.

Carbohydrate and protein require more steps in the digestion process than fats. That process causes your body to use more energy, which means it burns more calories than when digesting fats. High fat intake is more likely to go straight to fat storage than carbohydrate or protein. All three act as fuel sources for the working muscle; yet carbohydrate is the best. In following the recommendations set out in Section III, Smart Exercise, you will learn how to utilize body fat as a fuel source.

# IT GETS EASY QUICKLY

After a few weeks, you will know calorie and fat contents of all the foods you consume regularly by heart. And as time goes by, you will constantly be adding more to your mental list. Eventually, you will not need to count anything when you get to your desired body fat level (see page 66). If you have 50 pounds to lose, it may take you 50 weeks based on a pound per week. If you are creating a 7,000 calorie deficit per week, it will only take 25 weeks. If it is 10 pounds you want to lose, it may take 10 weeks or 5 weeks based on the 7,000 calorie deficit per week. I do not recommend losing more than 2 pounds per week. You will set yourself up for failure. About 95 percent of those who lose weight rapidly, gain it all back and in most cases they gain more.

# CHAPTER 11

## BIOLOGICAL THERMOSTAT?

If you have experienced the "ups and downs" of body fat fluxuations throughout your life, you have been re-setting your biological thermostat in an erratic fashion. These "ups and downs" are detrimental to your health. If you are fortyish now and have only gained ten pounds since your twentieth birthday, you have re-set your biological thermostat. Regardless of your weight gain and/or loss over the years, your thermostat is not broken. It constantly adapts to changes in body fat.

This chapter will be extremely helpful to you in, first, understanding your biological thermostat, and second, re-setting and maintaining it effortlessly for the rest of your life at a healthy body fat percentage (see page 66).

Those of you who have been on the "typical diet roller coaster" most likely have experienced the following physiological pitfalls.

**Weeks 1-4—Severe caloric restriction = dramatic weight loss.**
1. The body is losing water at a ratio much higher than it is losing fat.
2. The body adjusts to the "crisis" and adapts to conserve fat.
3. Muscle is burned along with fat to provide energy.

### Months 1-4—Weight loss slows and further progress becomes difficult.

1. Basal (resting) metabolic rate is significantly depressed.
2. Biological thermostat (setpoint) is being tampered with and is constantly trying to readjust all of your organ systems to your new weight.
3. Your organs begin to cry "mutiny," and some may actually do it.
4. Muscle tissue continues to be used as a fuel.
5. Nutritional deficiencies begin to show up in the form of weakness, fatigue, hair loss, thyroid problems, depression and others.

### By the end of the 4th month, the diet is discontinued and the weight is regained.

1. The satiety (feeling of fullness) center of the hypothalamus in the brain has been tampered with so much that it waits a long time to release cholecystokinin (CCK, the hormone that makes you feel full).
2. You go back to your old ways of eating because you're "sick and tired of being sick and tired" and all that food makes you feel good temporarily.
3. The higher setpoint (lowered metabolic rate) on your biological thermostat increases your body's tendency to put on more body fat because of the lost muscle. You may end up weighing the same as your pre-diet weight, but you have more fat and less muscle on your frame.

## DISPELLING THE 1,500 CALORIE MYTH

For you to be successful on this program, you need your own per-

38

sonal caloric intake numbers to go by. Fifteen hundred calories per day do not work for everyone as some have suggested, although it does work for a select few. It leaves heavier people hungry because they lose too much too fast. The 100 pound 20 percent body fat individuals who want to reduce to 12 percent end up putting on body fat at 1500 calories per day. *One size does not fit all* when it pertains to your caloric intake.

# CHAPTER 12

## BASAL METABOLIC RATE (BMR)

*Your intake numbers directly reflect your expenditure numbers.* If your intake is 1,560 calories per day and your expenditure is 1,560 calories per day, you will neither gain nor lose body fat. Most of us did a facsimile of that cycle through our teen years and twenties. Then we moved on to desk jobs and sedentary life styles coupled with the slowdown in growth hormone production, and we started "putting it on." The following list accounts for all of your daily sedentary activities (sleeping, getting out of bed, eating, sitting at your desk, walking to your car, driving it, computer tasks, having sex, talking on the phone, etc.). You burn calories every minute of the day. The table below represents your resting metabolic rate, or what some call your basal metabolic rate (BMR). I have added a factor to the BMR to account for all of our sedentary activities. You will use this number as your constant. If you weigh 150 pounds, your constant is 1,560 calories. As you lose weight to 145 pounds, your constant changes to 1,490. Let us say that you like your current weight of 150 pounds, and you walk briskly for an hour six days a week. You could consume your BMR of 1,560 + 400 (see exercise calorie chart on page 149), totaling 1,960 calories for each of those six days and not gain any body fat. You could consume only 1,560 calories on day

41

seven without gaining body fat since you do not walk on that day.

## MUSCLE IS METABOLICALLY ACTIVE, FAT IS NOT!

Your numbers are not always going to be exact. Researchers have known for years that caloric intake and expenditure numbers are just scientific guesses, but are the best tools we have. So if you are off 10 or 20 calories here or there, it is of minor concern. A muscular 150 pound lean body builder has a little higher BMR than a 150 pound over fat person. Most of us, however, are somewhere in between, which is what the numbers below estimate. You will find out how lean or over fat you are when you get to page 66. If you are lean and muscular, then you may want to add 100 calories or so to your BMR.

Mental calculations are much easier if you round numbers up or down. If your BMR is 930, use 900. If it is 860, use 900. If you have inadvertently misfigured a pound after a month or so, no big deal. Let us say that you run a cash register for a living and you are off $5 one way or the other after a month, there is no great concern. The next month when you are off $100, you become concerned. After the third month if you are off $500, your boss is seriously considering firing you. You get motivated quickly to find out what the problem is. Find it, make the adjustment, and all is well.

## YOUR BMR

**Table 12-1**

| Weight in pounds | BMR plus sedentary factor |
|:---:|:---:|
| 90 | 720 |
| 95 | 790 |

| Weight in pounds | BMR plus sedentary factor |
|---|---|
| 100 | 860 |
| 105 | 930 |
| 110 | 1,000 |
| 115 | 1,070 |
| 120 | 1,140 |
| 125 | 1,210 |
| 130 | 1,280 |
| 135 | 1,350 |
| 140 | 1,420 |
| 145 | 1,490 |
| 150 | 1,560 |
| 155 | 1,630 |
| 160 | 1,700 |
| 165 | 1,770 |
| 170 | 1,840 |
| 175 | 1,910 |
| 180 | 1,980 |
| 185 | 2,050 |
| 190 | 2,120 |
| 195 | 2,190 |
| 200 | 2,260 |
| 205 | 2,330 |
| 210 | 2,400 |
| 215 | 2,470 |
| 220 | 2,540 |
| 225 | 2,610 |
| 230 | 2,680 |
| 235 | 2,750 |
| 240 | 2,820 |
| 245 | 2,890 |
| 250 | 2,960 |
| 255 | 3,030 |
| 260 | 3,100 |
| 265 | 3,170 |
| 270 | 3,240 |
| 275 | 3,310 |
| 280 | 3,380 |

| Weight in pounds | BMR plus sedentary factor |
|:---:|:---:|
| 285 | 3,450 |
| 290 | 3,520 |
| 295 | 3,590 |
| 300 | 3,660 |

All of the BMR numbers are in increments of 70. If you weigh 85 pounds, take 70 calories from the 720 BMR for your constant. If you weigh 305 pounds, then add 70 to the 3,660 for your constant and so on.

# CHAPTER 13

## SHOULD I BE COUNTING FAT GRAMS ONLY?

**There are a couple of potential problems with counting fat grams.**
1. If you are limiting yourself to 30 grams of fat per day, you can find many foods with zero to one gram of fat. You begin to load up on these and eventually find that you are consuming 2,500-3,000 calories per day, equating to about 10 percent of the calories from fat.If you weigh 130 pounds and walk briskly for an hour per day (or any number of combinations), *you will put on body fat.* Either protein, carbohydrate, or fat consumed in excess of what your body is burning will be converted to and stored as body fat.

2. You may also selectively avoid buying a lot of your favorite foods because they say 10, 20, or 30 grams per serving. As that begins to happen, you start to feel deprived and revolt against the whole idea of losing body fat. I occasionally enjoy a couple of servings of Wavy Lay's (300 calories, 20 grams of fat), or 2 servings of pistachio nuts (380 calories, 28 grams of fat), as one of my five meals, and certainly do not feel guilty about it. Recall there are four other very low fat meals to bring the average percentage of calories from fat down.

# CHAPTER 14

## MAKE YOURSELF ACCOUNTABLE

There are many ways to keep track of daily caloric intake and expenditure numbers. Many clients use a wall calendar or appointment book to jot down their numbers. Others, including me, keep a mental running count and write the total down at bedtime. Some use the chart from page 51. In the beginning, it may be easier for you to jot down everything as you consume it. After awhile, you will be able to keep it in your head until bedtime. Many of us tend to cheat ourselves without realizing it. We will forget about a cookie or piece of candy that we had earlier because we get so busy with our everyday affairs. If it becomes a daily omission, it may discourage you after a month or so because the numbers can turn into pounds gained or pounds you are not losing. If that happens, check yourself a little closer.

## IN REALITY...

Your numbers may or may not go exactly according to plan...and that is okay. It is great to have an exact plan to go by, but we all have circumstances that throw a kink in "The Best Made Plans." Below (Table 14-1) is a sample month taken from my own calendar.

**Table 14-1.**

# January 1994

| Calories in | 1600[26] | 1200[27] | 1300[28] | 1500[29] | 1200[30] | 2200[31] | 3200 [1] | 2250 |
|---|---|---|---|---|---|---|---|---|
| Calories out | 1600 | 2550 | 2100 | 2500 | 2500 | 1600 | 1600 | weekly |
| | **0** | **-1350** | **-800** | **-1000** | **-1300** | **+600** | **+1600** | defecit |
| Calories in | 1700 [2] | 1200 [3] | 1400 [4] | 1500 [5] | 1800 [6] | 1700[7] | 3250 [8] | 5450 |
| Calories out | 2500 | 2300 | 2400 | 4000 | 2500 | 2150 | 2150 | weekly |
| | **-800** | **-1100** | **-1000** | **-2500** | **-700** | **-450** | **+1100** | defecit |
| Calories in | 3200 [9] | 1400[10] | 1450[11] | 3250[12] | 1350 [13] | 1600[14] | 2600[15] | 1700 |
| Calories out | 1600 | 2500 | 2300 | 2650 | 2400 | 2700 | 2400 | weekly |
| | **+1600** | **-1100** | **-850** | **+600** | **-1050** | **-1100** | **+200** | defecit |
| Calories in | 3300[16] | 1600[17] | 1500[18] | 1200[19] | 1600[20] | 3300[21] | 2700[22] | 3400 |
| Calories out | 2400 | 2700 | 2700 | 2900 | 2200 | 3200 | 2500 | weekly |
| | **+900** | **-1100** | **-1200** | **-1700** | **-600** | **+100** | **+200** | defecit |
| Calories in | 3000[23] | 1750[24] | 1950[25] | 1500[26] | 2600[27] | 2200[28] | 4200[29] | 1250 |
| Calories out | 2400 | 3450 | 1800 | 2600 | 3100 | 3200 | 1900 | weekly |
| | **+600** | **-1700** | **+150** | **-1100** | **-500** | **-1000** | **+2300** | defecit |

## 14050 Monthly deficit
### which equates to about 4 pounds of body fat!

My body fat was 12.9 percent on 12/26/93, and I weighed 154 pounds. On 1/29/95, my body fat was 10.2 percent, and I weighed 149 pounds. That equates to a 5 pound drop in weight and about a 3 percent drop in body fat. The following calculation is how it computes:

**154 minus 1 percent (1.54 pounds) = 152.46 pounds.**
**152.46 minus 1 percent (1.52 pounds) = 150.94 pounds.**
**150.94 minus 1 percent (1.51 pounds) = 149.43 pounds.**

48

Notice there are 13 of 35 days on which calorie consumption exceeds 2,000. The two days that show 2,200 *calories in* are not necessarily "pig out" days. "Piggin' out" represents high-calorie, high-fat consumption. 2,200 *calories in* does not necessarily represent high-calorie, high-fat consumption for someone this size. It is possible to have;

1. high-calorie, low-fat,
2. low-calorie, high-fat, and/or
3. low-calorie, low-fat.

In most instances, high-calorie consumption goes along with high-fat consumption. In this case, the two 2,200 calorie days were low in fat. Delete the two 2,200 calorie days from the 13 that exceed 2,000 calories, and that leaves 11 actual "pig out" days, amounting to more than two "pig out" days per week as previously stated. That is just how it happened to have worked out for that period of time. Sometimes I have less than two and sometimes more than two "pig out" days per week, but it averages out eventually.

The *calories out* numbers fluctuate because of the different amounts of exercise involved. My BMR was 1,600, even though the chart shows 1,560 for 150 pounders and 1,630 for 155 pounders. (To clarify my earlier statement on page 48 about my weight and BMR, I have since lost more body fat and gained more muscle accounting for the fact that I weigh 160 pounds at the time of this writing). It is much easier to round up or down when using big numbers: goals still get met. Also, notice how the *calories in* numbers can vary unless you are a little more disciplined as is my client Valerie, whose numbers are shown in the following calendar (Table 14-2).

Valerie's body fat measured 21.1 percent on 3/26/95, and she weighed 99 pounds. On 4/29/95, her body fat was 17.7 percent, and she weighed 98 pounds. There was a reduction of about 3 percent in body fat and only one pound in weight actually lost. It is common for body fat reduction not to match the actual weight loss. She gained a couple of pounds of muscle, the offsetting factor; and she looks much better as a result.

As your weight drops, if that is your desire, your BMR number will drop correspondingly. In Valerie's case, it stayed the same. I kept the same number because of the small amount of weight (five pounds) lost. For those of you who have higher amounts to lose, then you will need to adjust your BMR number downward periodically.

**Table 14-2**

## April 1995

| | | | | | | | |
|---|---|---|---|---|---|---|---|
| Calories in  900[26] | 900[27] | 900[28] | 900[29] | 900[30] | 1000[31] | 900[1] | **2200** |
| Calories out 1600 | 1200 | 1200 | 1350 | 1150 | 1200 | 900 | weekly |
| **-700** | **-300** | **-300** | **-450** | **-250** | **-200** | **0** | defecit |
| Calories in  900[2] | 900[3] | 950[4] | 900[5] | 950[6] | 1000[7] | 850[8] | **1200** |
| Calories out  900 | 1150 | 900 | 1250 | 1200 | 900 | 1350 | weekly |
| **0** | **-250** | **+50** | **-350** | **-250** | **+100** | **-500** | defecit |
| Calories in  950[9] | 950[10] | 1000[11] | 1000[12] | 800[13] | 1000[14] | 1000[15] | **1800** |
| Calories out  900 | 1000 | 1200 | 1300 | 1300 | 1300 | 1500 | weekly |
| **+50** | **-50** | **-200** | **-300** | **-500** | **-300** | **-500** | defecit |
| Calories in  900[16] | 1000[17] | 950[18] | 950[19] | 800[20] | 850[21] | 1000[22] | **1850** |
| Calories out 1150 | 1600 | 950 | 1050 | 1350 | 1350 | 900 | weekly |
| **-250** | **-600** | **+50** | **-100** | **-550** | **-500** | **+100** | defecit |
| Calories in  700[23] | 750[24] | 700[25] | 1000[26] | 800[27] | 900[28] | 800[29] | **3500** |
| Calories out 1150 | 1200 | 1500 | 1200 | 1200 | 1150 | 1750 | weekly |
| **-450** | **-450** | **-800** | **-200** | **-400** | **-250** | **-950** | defecit |

### 10550 Monthly deficit
### which equates to about 3 pounds of body fat!

# CHAPTER 15

## YOUR OWN LITTLE CALORIES IN AND OUT PAGE

Date_____

Name_____          Age_____

Weight_____

Body Fat Percentage (*see Chapter 17*) _____

| **Calories in**<br>(List numbers below) | **You ate what?**<br>(List below what<br>you ate each meal). | **%fat calories** |
| --- | --- | --- |

**Meal #1** _____  — — — — — — — — — — — — — — _____

*PLUS*

**Meal #2** _____  — — — — — — — — — — — — — — _____

*PLUS*

**Meal #3** _____ _ _ _ _ _ _ _ _ _ _ _ _ _ _ _ _____

*PLUS*

**Meal #4** _____ _ _ _ _ _ _ _ _ _ _ _ _ _ _ _ _____

*PLUS*

**Meal #5** _____ _ _ _ _ _ _ _ _ _ _ _ _ _ _ _____

**Your total number of calories for the day** _____

**Your total percentage of fat calories for the day** _____

*MINUS*

**Calories out** _____ Your BMR calories expended (see page 42) plus exercise calories expended (see page 149).

**Equals =** _____ **your deficit for the day!**

*You're so good....Congratulations!*

# CHAPTER 16

## REACTIVE EATING

Depression, boredom, and anger generally precipitate reactive eating. Keep a diary or note pad handy and write your feelings as you feel that an emotion is enticing you to consume mass quantities. You will find that eventually the desire for food will drop. Staying busy, exercising, and taking supplements will also contribute to the displacement of these feelings.

## STAY BUSY

Getting or staying involved in your faith, family activities, or job will keep your mind occupied with constructive things. If you do not have any of the above, do volunteer or charity work. Meals on Wheels, nursing home activities, or food serving lines are good examples of how you can make yourself busy while feeling great about yourself. These activities are very rewarding for you and for the ones you serve.

# FAST FOOD RESTAURANTS

As you stick with this plan, you will find that all the fast food restaurants become less and less desirable. As I have mentioned, I enjoy high-fat foods occasionally; but they are not as paramount on my mind as when they were my main fare. Most fast food restaurants now have nutrition information pamphlets that tell you calories per serving and fat grams and/or calories from fat. If it tells you only fat grams per serving, multiply the number of fat grams times nine to get the total calories from fat. Example: 10 fat grams times 9 equals 90 calories from fat. If the calories per serving is 270, the percentage of calories from fat is about 33 percent.

# DOOMED TO COUNT CALORIES FOREVER?

As you reach your desired body fat percentage, you can stop counting calories. Your biological thermostat takes over, and you will find that it is just as easy to maintain 10 percent body fat (if that is your goal) as it is 20 percent (assuming that was your original body fat percentage). I stopped counting calories 5/1/94 through 10/15/94. I kept the same eating, supplement, and exercise routine as always. My objective was to see if my biological thermostat would take over since I was not aware of my *calorie in* and *out* numbers. My body fat percentage varied from 8.3 to 9.2 percent during that time. For consistency, I measured and weighed myself each Saturday morning as soon as I got out of bed.

# CHAPTER 17

## HEIGHT/WEIGHT CHARTS?
## SKINFOLD CALIPERS? BATHROOM SCALES?

You can be considered "desirable," according to the height/weight charts, but be over-fat. You can be considered obese for your size, according to the same charts, yet carry only 5 percent body fat. These charts have been found to be inaccurate in more than 40 percent of all cases. Throw them away.

The most accurate way to keep track of your fat (50 percent or more is the layer of fat found just beneath the skin) is with a combination of skinfold calipers and a good set of scales (not the cheap bathroom scales). The technique of underwater weighing is as accurate or more than using skinfold calipers, yet it takes expensive equipment and is very time consuming. I recommend using the three-site method (discussed in the next few pages) with skinfold calipers because of ease, time, consistency, and self administration.

Measure and weigh yourself at least bi-weekly. If you see the millimeters of thickness on the skinfold calipers (page 56) start to rise, return to counting calories for as long as it takes to get yourself back down to your desired body fat. It is empowering to know that you have the ability to manipulate your body fat in this way.

Using scales as your only tool for body weight measurement, poses a couple of problems;

1. You may be losing fat while gaining muscle at the same time causing you to show weight gain, the same weight, or weight lost.

2. Water weighs about 8 pounds per gallon. Many people (of the heavier variety) can experience this 8 pound weight fluctuation in a day. That weight will show up on the scales and may either excite you (if you are dehydrated), or depress you (if you are hydrated). In this case, you lost weight (water only) but did not lose body fat. Skinfold measurements combined with weighing yourself is the way to go. In the case of Valerie, we were able to see a considerable drop in body fat along with just a 1 pound drop on the scales, telling us she lost fat while building muscle. How did I know it was not a water weight-loss concern? Because I measured and weighed her at the same time every week while she was following this program.

Below is a picture of the skinfold calipers that I use and recommend. They are much less expensive, just as accurate, and a lot easier to use than others on the market I have used.

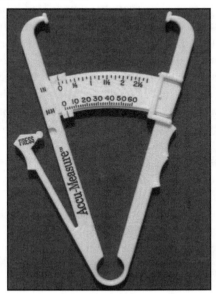

They can be purchased from Accu-Measure, Inc., 1-800-866-2727 (department D) for $19.95 plus shipping. They come with their own body fat interpretation chart. The calipers are great, but their chart says I would be at an "Ideal" body fat level in the range of about 14-21 percent. On me, 15 percent displays a protruding gut, large "love handles," and a fat face, which is okay for some but not for me. It also says the range of about 20-24 percent is "Ideal" for Valerie. She was not happy with thigh cellulite at 21.1 percent! I have measured thousands of people; and, in my opinion, these "Ideal" percentages would be better classified as "over-fat." The more fat you have on your body, the more likely you are to develop heart disease (kills about three quarter million people per year) and cancer (kills about half million people per year) among other diseases. The following charts (pages 62-65) and fatness rating scale (page 66) display healthy percentages for you to follow.

Another big reward for those of you who are concerned about your appearance is the unveiling of what some call the "six pack," "washboard," or "abs" (the muscles of the abdomen). We all have them; they just happen to be covered up by a thick layer of fat. They start becoming visible for most people in the 10 percent and below body fat range for men and the 15 percent and below range for women. There is no such thing as "spot reduction." Do not be led to believe that exercising your abs "till you're blue in the face" will make them surface. *The bottom line is body fat reduction.* When you lose body fat, you lose it from all parts of your body. Performing abdomen exercises makes the abs a bit bigger but burns an insignificant amount of calories compared to exercising large muscle groups (buttocks and legs).

I recommend the three-site measuring method for men and women. The front middle of the thigh is the only common site that men and women share. The following pictures show the sites and how to use the calipers.

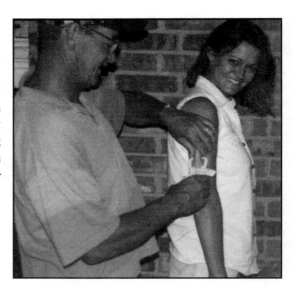

The first site on females is midway between the elbow joint and shoulder joint at the back middle of the upper arm.

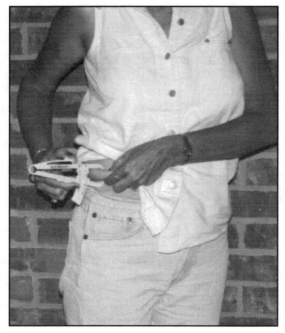

The second site is just above the iliac crest. It is the top of the hip bone on the side of your body.

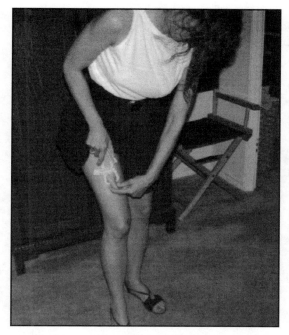

The third site is the front of the thigh midway between the knee joint and hip joint.

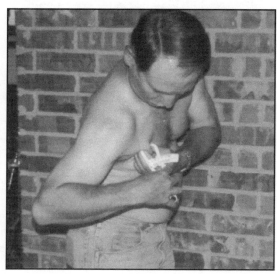

The first site for men is midway between the nipple and the joint of the shoulder.

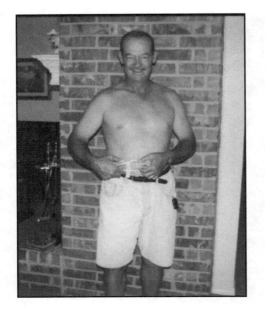

The second site is just to the side of the belly button.

The third site for males is the same as females: the front middle of the thigh midway between the knee joint and the hip joint. See the female thigh picture.

## CONSISTENCY IS THE KEY!

1. Always measure the same side of your body; do not combine or mix right side measurements with left side measurements.
2. Measure only skin, not through clothes.
3. Females may need a helper on the arm measurement site.
4. Relax the body part you are measuring to enable you to grab the fat.
5. Grab as big of a hunk as you can with your thumb and index finger.
6. Squeeze that hunk just shy of pain.
7. Place the caliper ends 1/4 of an inch away from your thumb and index

finger.

8. Squeeze the calipers together slowly around the fat (5 seconds) until the "press lever" clicks into place.

9. Measure each site several times until you read the same number (in millimeters) at least three times.

10. Females add the arm, hip bone, and thigh sites together.

11. Males add the chest, belly button, and thigh sites together.

12. Take the sum of your measurements and look on the following chart for your body fat percentage under your gender and age.

**Table 17-1**

# CHART FOR MEN

Percent fat estimates for men: sum of chest, abdominal, and thigh skin folds.

| Sum of Skin Folds (mm) | AGE TO THE LAST YEAR | | | | | | | | |
|---|---|---|---|---|---|---|---|---|---|
| | Under 22 | 23-27 | 28-32 | 33-37 | 38-42 | 43-47 | 48-52 | 53-57 | Over 58 |
| 8-10 | 1.3 | 1.8 | 2.3 | 2.9 | 3.4 | 3.9 | 4.5 | 5.0 | 5.5 |
| 11-13 | 2.2 | 2.8 | 3.3 | 3.9 | 4.4 | 4.9 | 5.5 | 6.0 | 6.5 |
| 14-16 | 3.2 | 3.8 | 4.3 | 4.8 | 5.4 | 5.9 | 6.4 | 7.0 | 7.5 |
| 17-19 | 4.2 | 4.7 | 5.3 | 5.8 | 6.3 | 6.9 | 7.4 | 8.0 | 8.5 |
| 20-22 | 5.1 | 5.7 | 6.2 | 6.8 | 7.3 | 7.9 | 8.4 | 8.9 | 9.5 |
| 23-25 | 6.1 | 6.6 | 7.2 | 7.7 | 8.3 | 8.8 | 9.4 | 9.9 | 10.5 |
| 26-28 | 7.0 | 7.6 | 8.1 | 8.7 | 9.2 | 9.8 | 10.3 | 10.9 | 11.4 |
| 29-31 | 8.0 | 8.5 | 9.1 | 9.6 | 10.2 | 10.7 | 11.3 | 11.8 | 12.4 |
| 32-34 | 8.9 | 9.4 | 10.0 | 10.5 | 11.1 | 11.6 | 12.2 | 12.8 | 13.3 |
| 35-37 | 9.8 | 10.4 | 10.9 | 11.5 | 12.0 | 12.6 | 13.1 | 13.7 | 14.3 |
| 38-40 | 10.7 | 11.3 | 11.8 | 12.4 | 12.9 | 13.5 | 14.1 | 14.6 | 15.2 |
| 41-43 | 11.6 | 12.2 | 12.7 | 13.3 | 13.8 | 14.4 | 15.0 | 15.5 | 16.1 |
| 44-46 | 12.5 | 13.1 | 13.6 | 14.2 | 14.7 | 15.3 | 15.9 | 16.4 | 17.0 |
| 47-49 | 13.4 | 13.9 | 14.5 | 15.1 | 15.6 | 16.2 | 16.8 | 17.3 | 17.9 |
| 50-52 | 14.3 | 14.8 | 15.4 | 15.9 | 16.5 | 17.1 | 17.6 | 18.2 | 18.8 |
| 53-55 | 15.1 | 15.7 | 16.2 | 16.8 | 17.4 | 17.9 | 18.5 | 19.1 | 19.7 |
| 56-58 | 16.0 | 16.5 | 17.1 | 17.7 | 18.2 | 18.8 | 19.4 | 20.0 | 20.5 |
| 59-61 | 16.9 | 17.4 | 17.9 | 18.5 | 19.1 | 19.7 | 20.2 | 20.8 | 21.4 |
| 62-64 | 17.6 | 18.2 | 18.8 | 19.4 | 19.9 | 20.5 | 21.1 | 21.7 | 22.2 |
| 65-67 | 18.5 | 19.0 | 19.6 | 20.2 | 20.8 | 21.3 | 21.9 | 22.5 | 23.1 |
| 68-70 | 19.3 | 19.9 | 20.4 | 21.0 | 21.6 | 22.2 | 22.7 | 23.3 | 23.9 |
| 71-73 | 20.1 | 20.7 | 21.2 | 21.8 | 22.4 | 23.0 | 23.6 | 24.1 | 24.7 |
| 74-76 | 20.9 | 21.5 | 22.0 | 22.6 | 23.2 | 23.8 | 24.4 | 25.0 | 25.5 |
| 77-79 | 21.7 | 22.2 | 22.8 | 23.4 | 24.0 | 24.6 | 25.2 | 25.8 | 26.3 |
| 80-82 | 22.4 | 23.0 | 23.6 | 24.2 | 24.8 | 25.4 | 25.9 | 26.5 | 27.1 |
| 83-85 | 23.2 | 23.8 | 24.4 | 25.0 | 25.5 | 26.1 | 26.7 | 27.3 | 27.9 |
| 86-88 | 24.0 | 24.5 | 25.1 | 25.7 | 26.3 | 26.9 | 27.5 | 28.1 | 28.7 |
| 89-91 | 24.7 | 25.3 | 25.9 | 25.5 | 27.1 | 27.6 | 28.2 | 28.8 | 29.4 |
| 92-94 | 25.4 | 26.0 | 26.6 | 27.2 | 27.8 | 28.4 | 29.0 | 29.6 | 30.2 |

| Sum of Skin Folds (mm) | AGE TO THE LAST YEAR | | | | | | | | |
|---|---|---|---|---|---|---|---|---|---|
| | Under 22 | 23-27 | 28-32 | 33-37 | 38-42 | 43-47 | 48-52 | 53-57 | Over 58 |
| 92-97 | 26.1 | 16.7 | 27.3 | 27.9 | 28.5 | 29.1 | 29.7 | 30.3 | 30.9 |
| 98-100 | 26.9 | 27.4 | 28.0 | 28.6 | 29.2 | 29.8 | 30.4 | 31.0 | 31.6 |
| 101-103 | 27.5 | 28.1 | 28.7 | 29.3 | 29.9 | 30.5 | 31.1 | 31.7 | 32.3 |
| 104-106 | 28.2 | 28.8 | 29.4 | 30.0 | 30.6 | 31.2 | 31.8 | 32.4 | 33.0 |
| 107-109 | 28.9 | 29.5 | 30.1 | 30.7 | 31.3 | 31.9 | 32.5 | 33.1 | 33.7 |
| 110-112 | 29.6 | 30.2 | 30.8 | 31.4 | 32.0 | 32.6 | 33.2 | 33.8 | 34.4 |
| 113-115 | 30.2 | 30.8 | 31.4 | 32.0 | 32.6 | 33.2 | 33.8 | 34.5 | 35.1 |
| 116-118 | 30.9 | 31.5 | 32.1 | 32.7 | 33.3 | 33.9 | 34.5 | 35.1 | 35.7 |
| 119-121 | 31.5 | 32.1 | 32.7 | 33.3 | 33.9 | 34.5 | 35.1 | 35.7 | 36.4 |
| 122-124 | 32.1 | 32.7 | 33.3 | 33.9 | 34.5 | 35.1 | 35.8 | 36.4 | 37.0 |
| 125-127 | 32.7 | 33.3 | 33.9 | 34.5 | 35.1 | 35.8 | 36.4 | 37.0 | 37.6 |

Percent fat calculated by the formula of Siri, W. "The Gross Composition of the Body." In: Lawrence, J. and Tobias, C. (editors), *Advances in Biological and Medical Physics*. 1956, Academic Press, New York.

Jackson, A. and Pollack, M. "Practical Assessment of Body Composition." *The Physician and Sports Medicine*. May, 1985, 13:86.

**Table 17-2**

## CHART FOR WOMEN

Percent fat estimates for women: sum of triceps, iliac crest, and thigh skin folds

| Sum of Skin Folds (mm) | AGE TO THE LAST YEAR | | | | | | | | |
|---|---|---|---|---|---|---|---|---|---|
| | Under 22 | 23-27 | 28-32 | 33-37 | 38-42 | 43-47 | 48-52 | 53-57 | Over 58 |
| 23-25 | 9.7 | 9.9 | 10.2 | 10.4 | 10.7 | 10.9 | 11.2 | 11.4 | 11.7 |
| 26-28 | 11.0 | 11.2 | 11.5 | 11.7 | 12.0 | 12.3 | 12.5 | 12.7 | 13.0 |
| 29-31 | 12.3 | 12.5, | 12.8 | 13.0 | 13.3 | 13.5 | 13.8 | 14.0 | 14.3 |
| 32-34 | 13.6 | 13.8 | 14.0 | 14.3 | 14.5 | 14.8 | 15.0 | 15.3 | 15.5 |
| 35-37 | 14.8 | 15.0 | 15.3 | 15.5 | 15.8 | 16.0 | 16.3 | 16.5 | 16.8 |
| 38-40 | 16.0 | 16.3 | 16.5 | 16.7 | 17.0 | 17.2 | 17.5 | 17.7 | 18.0 |
| 41-43 | 17.2 | 17.4 | 17.7 | 17.9 | 18.2 | 18.4 | 18.7 | 18.9 | 19.2 |
| 44-46 | 18.3 | 18.6 | 18.8 | 19.1 | 19.3 | 19.6 | 19.8 | 20.1 | 20.3 |
| 47-49 | 19.5 | 19.7 | 20.0 | 20.2 | 20.5 | 20.7 | 21.0 | 21.2 | 21.5 |
| 50-52 | 20.6 | 20.8 | 21.1 | 21.3 | 21.6 | 21.8 | 22.1 | 22.3 | 22.6 |
| 53-55 | 21.7 | 21.9 | 22.1 | 22.4 | 22.6 | 22.9 | 23.1 | 23.4 | 23.6 |
| 56-58 | 22.7 | 23.0 | 23.2 | 23.4 | 23.7 | 23.9 | 24.2 | 24.4 | 24.7 |
| 59-61 | 23.7 | 24.0 | 24.2 | 24.5 | 24.7 | 25.0 | 25.2 | 25.5 | 25.7 |
| 62-64 | 24.7 | 25.0 | 25.2 | 25.5 | 25.7 | 26.0 | 26.7 | 26.4 | 26.7 |
| 65-67 | 25.7 | 25.9 | 26.2 | 26.4 | 26.7 | 26.9 | 27.2 | 27.4 | 27.7 |
| 68-70 | 26.6 | 26.9 | 27.1 | 27.4 | 27.6 | 27.9 | 28.1 | 28.4 | 28.6 |
| 71-73 | 27.5 | 27.8 | 28.0 | 28.3 | 28.5 | 28.8 | 28.0 | 29.3 | 29.5 |
| 74-76 | 28.4 | 28.7 | 28.9 | 29.2 | 29.4 | 29.7 | 29.9 | 30.2 | 30.4 |
| 77-79 | 29.3 | 29.5 | 29.8 | 30.0 | 30.3 | 30.5 | 30.8 | 31.0 | 31.3 |
| 80-82 | 30.1 | 30.4 | 30.6 | 30.9 | 31.1 | 31.4 | 31.6 | 31.9 | 32.1 |
| 83-85 | 30.9 | 31.2 | 31.4 | 31.7 | 31.9 | 32.2 | 32.4 | 32.7 | 32.9 |
| 86-88 | 31.7 | 32.0 | 32.2 | 32.5 | 32.7 | 32.9 | 33.2 | 33.4 | 33.7 |
| 89-91 | 32.5 | 32.7 | 33.0 | 33.2 | 33.5 | 33.7 | 33.9 | 34.2 | 34.4 |
| 92-94 | 33.2 | 33.4 | 33.7 | 33.9 | 34.2 | 34.4 | 34.7 | 34.9 | 35.2 |
| 95-97 | 33.9 | 34.1 | 34.4 | 34.6 | 34.9 | 35.1 | 35.4 | 35.6 | 35.9 |
| 98-100 | 34.6 | 34.8 | 35.1 | 35.3 | 35.5 | 35.8 | 36.0 | 36.3 | 36.5 |
| 101-103 | 35.3 | 35.4 | 35.7 | 35.9 | 36.2 | 36.4 | 36.7 | 36.9 | 37.2 |
| 104-106 | 35.8 | 36.1. | 36.3 | 36.6 | 36.8 | 37.1 | 37.3 | 37.5 | 37.8 |
| 107-109 | 36.4 | 36.7 | 36.9 | 37.1 | 37.4 | 37.6 | 37.9 | 38.1 | 38.4 |

| Sum of Skin Folds (mm) | AGE TO THE LAST YEAR | | | | | | | | |
|---|---|---|---|---|---|---|---|---|---|
| | Under 22 | 23-27 | 28-32 | 33-37 | 38-42 | 43-47 | 48-52 | 53-57 | Over 58 |
| 110-112 | 37.0 | 37.2 | 37.5 | 37.7 | 38.0 | 38.2 | 38.5 | 38.7 | 38.9 |
| 113-115 | 37.5 | 37.8 | 38.0 | 38.2 | 38.5 | 38.7 | 39.0 | 39.2 | 39.5 |
| 116-118 | 38.0 | 38.3 | 38.5 | 38.8 | 39.0 | 39.3 | 39.5 | 39.7 | 40.0 |
| 119-121 | 38.5 | 38.7 | 39.0 | 39.2 | 39.5 | 39.7 | 40.0 | 40.2 | 40.5 |
| 122-124 | 39.0 | 39.2 | 39.4 | 39.7 | 39.9 | 40.2 | 40.4 | 40.7 | 40.9 |
| 125-127 | 39.4 | 39.6 | 39.9 | 40.1 | 40.4 | 40.6 | 40.9 | 41.1 | 41.4 |
| 128-130 | 39.8 | 40.0 | 40.3 | 40.5 | 40.8 | 41.0 | 41.3 | 41.5 | 41.8 |

Percent fat calculated by the formula of Siri, W. "The Gross Composition of the Body." In: Lawrence, J. and Tobias, C. (editors), *Advances in Biological and Medical Physics*. 1956, Academic Press, NewYork.

Jackson, A. and Pollack, M. "Practical Assessment of Body Composition." *The Physician and Sports Medicine*. May, 1985, 13:86.

**Table 17-3**

## BODY FAT PERCENTAGE RATING SCALE

| Classification | Men% | Women% |
|---|---|---|
| • Very Lean "World Class Athletes"<br>(heart and other disease rates virtually non-existent) | 2-8 | 5-10 |
| • Lean<br>(a little better chance for developing heart and other diseases) | 9-12 | 11-14 |
| • Less Lean<br>(you are a little pudgy!) | 13-15 | 15-18 |
| • Far From Lean<br>(heart and other disease rates significantly higher) | 16-above | 19-above |

# CHAPTER 18

## "IT'S SOMETHIN' IN THE WATER!"

Our tap water and many bottled waters are full of contamanants. Viruses, bacteria, pesticides, herbicides, fertilizers, asbestos fibers (not a good way to get your daily fiber), chlorine, radioactive wastes, arsenic, soap, wood pulp, oil, sulfuric acid, copper, paint, and other chemicals from industry too numerous to mention are just some of the things that show up in our water supplies.

Chlorine is an oxidizing agent added to our water supplies. It was used in World War I to kill people, and it still is. Combined with animal fats in our diet, it becomes a sticky paste-like substance that adheres to our artery walls, causing heart disease. Trihalomethanes, a by-product of chlorine, is a known contributor to liver, bladder, and colorectal cancer.

Oxidizing agents are related to the destructive free radical activity that goes on inside of us and all around us. It is the unpaired oxygen molecule that cannot find a mate, becomes angry, and destroys everything it can to find that mate. The unified theory of aging and disease is the product of this free radical ordeal as discovered in the late 1950's by Dr. Denham Harman of the University of Nebraska. In our bodies, the results of this activity are arthritis, cancer, heart disease, etc. Externally, a rusted out car, a rotting banana, peroxidized hamburger meat, etc. become victims of free radical activity.

Government figures estimate that about 900,000 people get sick from U.S.A. water laced with harmful bacteria.

Approximately 55,000 of the regulated chemical dumps in the U.S.A. are leaking into the water table.

There are approximately 200,000 illegal, unregulated chemical dumps in the U.S.A. leaking into the water table.

The EPA in 1993 reported that 819 water systems in the U.S.A. had toxic levels of lead in fully treated water.

There are about 60,000 different chemicals in our water supplies of which the treatment stations can afford only to test for 30-40 of them. That leaves more than 59,000.

## LET'S CLEAN IT UP!

The way to measure water for contaminants is by parts per million (ppm). Typical faucet water can have 250-1,000 ppm contaminants. We ideally want it to be zero ppm. Getting to zero is elusive. The Colgan Institute in California reports that distillation can bring tap water down to 2-12 ppm. The reverse osmosis process is just as good as distillation, and that is about as good as it gets. Bottled distilled and bottled reverse osmosis treated water is good, also. Bottled mineral and drinking water is not good unless it says distilled or has been put through reverse osmosis. Read the label the next time you pick up a bottle of expensive bottled water. Ionization and carbon filtering are not very good either. Remember the multi-level company that sold the carbon filtering device

68

for $300-$500?  Beware!

A more cost effective way to buy water is from a water store or purchase a distillation or reverse osmosis unit for your home.  Pure Water, Inc. of Lincoln, Nebraska 402-467-9300 sells distillation units and Water Event in the Dallas/Fort Worth, Texas area 1-800-232-3330 sells reverse osmosis units.


## DRINK IT WISELY

I have read throughout the years from various sources that we all should drink eight glasses of water per day.  A glass to me is about 20 ounces; 20 times 8 is 160 ounces, a quart shy of a gallon and a half per day.  A glass to you may be 8 ounces.  8 times 8 is 64 ounces.  That is a big discrepancy.  As a result, I never knew how much water to drink.  After experimenting with water consumption over the years, and relieving myself from every 30 minutes or so, to  every 5 hours or so, I discovered that every 3 hours is optimum.  There are many factors involved in the amount of water consumption that will make you urinate every three hours; mainly heat, humidity, exercise, and body size.  As these factors change, your water consumption will change.  I suggest you experiment for yourself in the same way as above to find out the amount of consumption that works for you.  As bedtime nears, back your consumption down so you do not have to get up in the middle of the night to urinate.


## ARE YOU DEHYDRATED?

Most of us are chronically dehydrated.  Problems ranging from low back pain, to constipation, to headaches, can be causative factors for low water intake.  Many of us were raised on sodas and fruit juices to satisfy our thirst.  Even though these have a high water content, they will not meet your need for water intake. They may even cause other health problems.

We are already dehydrated if we depend on thirst as the signal to drink. The amount you consume depends on many factors as mentioned above. A dehydrated muscle can mean a 10 percent loss of strength and 8 percent loss of speed. That loss can be the difference between first and last in athletic competition.

Water retention will become a thing of the past as you increase your consumption. Just like fat, the body is finally letting go of what it is being starved of. As you feed your body five meals per day, the body does not perceive the threat of starvation and releases fat more readily for fuel. The same happens with water, although it is used for cooling and hydration and helps rid the body of wastes. The stress on the liver and kidneys is alleviated; and they; in turn; are more efficient at processing fats and expelling wastes respectively.

## HUNGER CAN BE THIRST IN DISGUISE

We have been misled to believe all of our lives that we should be consuming soft drinks, beer, sport drinks, etc., to satisfy our thirst. They can and do to a certain degree, yet the repercussions can be severe dehydration (anything with alcohol in it), and or the accumulation of fat. Anything (carbohydrate, fat, and protein) consumed in excess of what you burn turns into fat.

Hydrate in the word carbohydrate refers to water. Generally, carbohydrates have the highest water content of all the foods we eat. Most of us are constantly trying to satisfy our thirst with foods. Unconsciencously, we are consuming lots of calories when we could be consuming none. I have many clients who have followed this pattern all of their lives. Drinking soft drinks, fruit juices, milk, and more is typical, not to mention "piggin' out" on solid foods all of the time to satisfy the thirst urge. Each time you feel hungry, try water instead, and make it part of your everyday fare. You will be pleasantly surprised as you start changing this part of your lifestyle.

# Section II

# *Smart*
# *Supplements*

# CHAPTER 19

## SMART SUPPLEMENTS

This section provides information about the best combinations of pharmaceutical grade supplements I have found. Each of them contains the amounts of every vitamin, mineral, amino acid, enzyme, and herb (VMAAEH) that scientific literature advocates, as close as any formula can. These supplements are the most cost effective in the world per gram. You will not find them in your grocery or drug store, but you may find a select few in a health food store with very high price tags, such as Twin Lab products.

This is my own independent study. I am not paid to endorse the supplements below, they just happen to have the best amounts and combinations I have found.

**LEM** stands for Life Extension Mix that can be obtained from the mail order company **Prolongevity, 1-800-841-5433**. This company charges a $75 per year membership fee, which pays for your first $75 worth of product and a subscription to the monthly magazine called Life Extension. The magazine includes research about supplements and other life saving therapies from around the world. Call for a price list or quotes on the products you are interested in.

There are other companies offering **pharmaceutical grade** products that are also in line with the recommendations, according to the scientific literature. You may want to check them out. They are **(1) Twin Lab through L & H Vitamins, 1-800-221-1152, (2) Vitamin Research Products, 1-800-877-2447, (3) Health Maintenance Programs, 1-800-362-8673, (4) Life Services Supplements, 1-800-542-3230, and (5) Healthy Directions, Inc., 1-800-722-8008.**

**Units of measurement for supplements are as follows:**
**International Unit (IU)** - Measures biological activity or potency, which is different from weight measurements shown below. IU is used for fat-soluble vitamins A, D, E, and K.
**Grams (gm.)** - Weight measurement: 1/28th of an ounce.
**Milligrams (mg.)** - 1/1000 of a gram.
**Micrograms (mcg.)** - 1/1000 of a milligram.

| Females 18 years of age and older | Males 18 years of age and older |
|---|---|
| **LEM** - 3 tablets every 5-6 hours = 9 total per day.<br>Build up to it if you are just starting out or if you have been off awhile.<br>1 tablet every 5-6 hours the first week.<br>2 tablets every 5-6 hours the second week.<br>3 tablets every 5-6 hours the third week until forever.<br>This formula comes *with or without extra niacin.* See vitamin B3, page 89 for more information.<br>The 40 plus nutrients in LEM and amounts of each | Same |

| Females 18 years of age and older | Males 18 years of age and older |
|---|---|
| are discussed completely in Chapter 20 based on the consumption of 9 tablets per day. | |
| **Extension Calcium** (Vitamin Research Products) 8-10 capsules per day. 2 capsules with the first LEM dose, 2 with the second dose, and 4-6 with the last dose (also see page 96). | 6-8 capsules per day. 1 capsule with the first LEM dose, 1 with the second, and 4-6 with the last. |
| **Extra Zinc**- 25-50 mg. per day (also see page 93). | Same |
| **Extra Vitamin C** - 1,000 - 15,000 mg. per day divided by three doses (this will make your total C intake 4,000-18,000 mg. because of the approximate 3,000 mg. in LEM). Also see page 84. | Same |
| **Extra Chromium Picolinate** - 200 mcg. (not mg.) per day. Also see page 97. | Same |

Most of the above supplements can be purchased from any of the other companies listed above other than Extension Calcium (Vitamin Research Products) and LEM (Prolongevity).

Prolongevity also has a good multi-VMAAEH formula for kids.
*Be sure to take all of the above with food and water (preferably distilled water or water that has been filtered through the process of reverse osmosis—see page 68).*
I recommend the full LEM plus 400-800 mcg. (not mg.) of folic acid and the above doses of calcium, magnesium, zinc, vitamin C, and chromium picolinate *for women during pregnancy.* Twinlab also has a liquid infant formula. Studies have shown that *sudden infant death syndrome* may be related to vitamin deficiencies, particularly biotin, vitamins C, and B1.

## PILL ORGANIZER

Pictured below is the best pill organizer box I have found. It can be purchased from The Container Store.

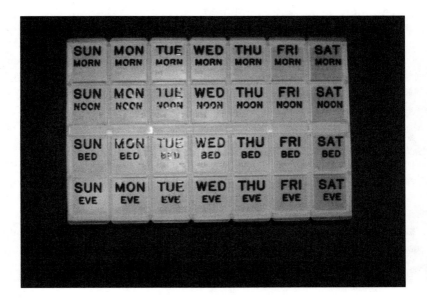

78

# SLOWLY BUILD UP WITH CONSISTENCY

Your body has to get used to the VMAAEHs gradually. It has never had this many tools (VMAAEHs) to work with before. It needs time to sort them all out. Compare the processes the body has to go through to your being introduced to forty plus new friends at a party one evening and being asked to get to know them all intimately by midnight. You would "freak out." Do not "freak out" your body.

Most VMAAEHs are water soluble. Soon after you consume the supplements, you slowly lose them through respiration, sweat, defecation, and urination. You can experiment for yourself. Take 50 mg. of vitamin B2 and watch your urine turn bright yellow within the next hour. A few hours later it will begin to fade. The blood and other body parts absorb and utilize what they need and send the rest along the excretory organs as it continues its functions. As you continue to take it throughout the day, your urine will maintain the bright yellow color. Skip a dose or two and you will see it fade again.

Even though you are slowly losing them, certain amounts of each supplement are remaining in your body. It is for this reason that you take them at least three times per day. Some researchers even advocate four times per day to maintain a consistently high blood (serum) level and to keep your excretory organs healthy as well. Our serum levels and body tissues eventually become saturated with each one. If you forget a dose, your serum level drops somewhat and makes you more susceptible to viral infection and disease. If you forget two or more doses in a row, then you are really asking for trouble. If you do contract a virus or disease, put yourself back on schedule as soon as possible and take some of the other supplements mentioned later in addition to your regular schedule of supplements.

If you decide to discontinue use of any supplements for any reason, taper off gradually. The body has to make metabolic adjustments just as it has to make the same adjustments as you are gradually increasing dosages. For example, if you abruptly stop taking vitamin C (more than a gram per day), you may experience subclinical symptoms of scurvy (a defiency syndrome of vitamin C).

## Of Greater Performance

As you become "supplement smart," you will most likely experience enhanced moods, have more energy, and wield better mental awareness. It is easy to understand why. You now have access to the best nutritional tools backed by scientific evidence. Our ancestors had access without scientific evidence through untampered food supplies.

## Recommended Daily Allowances — A Good Smoke Screen

The amounts of each supplement you will be consuming will be much greater than the Recommended Daily Allowances (RDAs). The RDAs are set by the Food and Nutrition Board (FNB-an arm of our government). The FNB ascertains these amounts mostly by seeing what is in our foods and concluding, that is the amount we need. These amounts are a far cry from what our bodies need to function properly. If we follow the RDAs, we are placing ourselves "on the edge of a fence" from which we can easily fall off into deficiency diseases. Actually, the RDAs are good for food manufacturers who like to boast that a serving of their food meets 100 percent of the RDAs of several vitamins and minerals. The FNB does not recognize many needed supplements such as chromium, selenium, potassium, grape seed extract, choline, taurine, and the list goes on. They contend that 60 mg. of vitamin C is sufficient to keep us free from viral infection and disease, an assertion that is simply not true.

## Like....Let's Get Elemental Man

Minerals listed on almost all labels are combined with a compound that delivers or makes the mineral better absorbed into the body. Using calcium as an example, it may be listed as calcium carbonate, calcium citrate, calcium stearate, and the list goes on. The LEM label says:

| | | |
|---|---|---|
| **Calcium citrate** | **500 mg.** | **10 percent of the RDA.** |
| **Calcium stearate** | **250 mg.** | **1.65 percent of the RDA.** |

The RDA for calcium is 1,200 mg. 10 percent of 1,200 equals 120. 1.65 percent of 1,200 is 19.8. 120 plus 19.8 equals 139.8. The nine pills per day of LEM will provide you with only 139.8 mg. of calcium, precisely the reason that I recommend extra minerals (*Extension Calcium*) on page 77. The above amounts are typical of how most minerals are listed on labels. 139.8 is the actual "elemental" amount of calcium or amount the body is getting and using. The *Extension Calcium* label shows the amount of calcium (1,000 mg. per six capsules) derived from calcium citrate (600 mg.) and calcium hydroxyapatite (400 mg). In contrast to the LEM label, the 1,000 mg. in this instance is the elemental amount. *Studies show that males require at least 1,200 elemental mg. per day and in contrast to the RDA above, females 18 years of age and older require 1,800 elemental mg. per day.*

Following my recommendations on page 77 and eating the foods covered in Section I will keep you safe from mineral deficiency diseases. There are more than 100 arthritis related diseases associated with mineral deficiencies with names like bursitis, rheumatism, tendinitis, pica, periodontitis, osteoarthritis, low back pain, and the list goes on. I hear regularly from clients who report solutions to health problems like the ones above after consuming the amounts recommended above.

# CHAPTER 20

## STUFF THAT MIRACLES ARE MADE OF

The amounts of VMAAEHs given below are the parts that make up the complete LEM formulation. Each nutrient has its own independent body of research. I received no help from Prolongevity or any other company financially or otherwise in the substantiation of the claims I have made below. *The amounts of each nutrient listed throughout Chapter 20 are from consuming 9 tablets per day.* Prolongevity has a powder and capsule form also. The amount of powder or number of capsules consumed will be different from the 9 tablets consumed. I have listed each one in the order it appears on the label.

## THE VEGETABLE OR CAROTENOID COMPLEX

**Beta carotene (25,000 IU); lycopene (tomato extract), (300 mg.); leutein (xanthophyll), (700 mg.); broccoli concentrate (200 mg.); cabbage concentrate (500 mg.); carrot powder (200 mg.); and tomato powder (200 mg.)** are invaluable to our nurtritional health. For decades, studies keep showing us that the carotenoids are very effective at anti-infection, cancer protection, immunity enhancement, fighting skin disorders such as acne and psoriasis along with zinc, preventing or reversing skin aging, speeding up the healing process of wounds, fighting atherosclerosis (blockages formed on the inside of artery walls causing heart attacks), being an internal sunscreen, and alleviating the side effects of radiation therapy.

## ASCORBATE-CITRUS ANTIOXIDANT COMPLEX

**Vitamin C, from calcium, magnesium, and niacinamide ascorbates (1,250 mg.); ascorbic acid (1,250 mg.); ascorbyl palmitate—fat soluble (500 mg.), and acerola juice powder (300 mg.)** is the everything vitamin. The first clinical experiment dates back to the 1750's when a British doctor put limes, which for foodstuffs are rich in vitamin C, in the rations of a group of sailors and compared this group to another group that received the same rations but without limes. The limeless group developed scurvy (wounds would not heal, gums bled, skin was rough, and muscles shrank). The lime group did not get scurvy and became known as "limeys" because they took limes with them on long voyages.

Robert Fulton Cathcart III, M.D., has had more clinical experience with vitamin C than probably anyone else. In the early 1970's, after reading Linus Pauling's book, *Vitamin C and the Common Cold,* he succeeded in treating inner ear and respiratory infections he had had since childhood with vitamin C. It was about that time that he decided to give up his practice as an orthopedic surgeon and become a general practitioner concerned with infectious diseases and their relationship to varying doses of vitamin C. By 1981, he was able to report his observations on 9,000 patients he treated with vitamin C.

Like so many of the other vitamins, it is water soluble (your body does not store it for very long). We can increase the blood levels by taking it throughout the day everyday. Dr. Cathcart found that we all have a bowel tolerance limit of vitamin C (the onset of diarrhea). His patients who had very low blood levels of vitamin C (the severely ill) could tolerate more than 200 gm. (not mg.) per day before the onset of diarrhea. As the patients' illnesses improved, the amount of vitamin C could be lowered because of the increased levels of it in the blood (serum level). The amount would then be lowered toward the normal 4-15 gm. per day range.

Your bowel tolerance limit is your barometer of vitamin C intake if you happen to contract any of the conditions listed below. Of course, water consumption (distilled or reverse osmosis; see page 68 for amounts) is highly recommended, even if you do not induce diarrhea with vitamin C. Soft drinks and coffee provide water but add calories, caffeine, sugar, and an acid pH. Most foods have water content as do fruit juices but, because of the extra calories, do not rely on them to quench your thirst.

**Table 20-1**

*The following table is what Dr. Cathcart developed, based on his research of vitamin C intake.*

| Condition | Grams/24 hours | Doses/24 hours |
|---|---|---|
| Normal | 4-15 | 4 |
| Mild cold | 30-60 | 6-10 |
| Severe cold | 60-100 | 8-15 |
| Influenza | 100-150 | 8-20 |
| ECH0, coxsackievirus | 100-150 | 8-20 |
| Mononucleosis | 150-200+ | 12-25 |
| Viral pneumonia | 100-200+ | 12-25 |
| Hayfever, asthma | 15-50 | 4-8 |
| Environmental and food allergy | 0.5-50 | 4-8 |
| Burn, injury, surgery | 25-150 | 6-20 |
| Anxiety, exercise,and other stress | 15-25 | 4-6 |
| Cancer | 15-100 | 4-15 |

| Condition | Grams/24 hours | Doses/24 hours |
|---|---|---|
| Ankylosing spondylitis | 15-100 | 4-15 |
| Reiter's syndrome | 15-60 | 4-10 |
| Acute anterior uveitis | 30-100 | 4-15 |
| Rheumatoid arthritis | 15-100 | 4-15 |
| Bacterial infections | 30-200+ | 10-25 |
| Infectious hepatitis | 30-100 | 6-15 |
| Candida infections | 15-200+ | 6-25 |

Dr. Cathcart's success has been replicated many times over in studies done by *Linus Pauling, Ewan Cameron, Irwin Stone*, and many others.

The above chart from *Medical Hypothesis*, 1981, 7:1359-1376 used by permission.

**Citrus bioflavonoids (250 mg.) and hesperidin complex (250 mg.)** are found in the colored parts of plants and white part of the inner orange peel. They strengthen capillaries, reduce inflammation, speed healing in ulcers, help in overcoming allergies, are anti-viral, inhibit the formation of prostaglandins (hormone-like compounds manufactured from essential fatty acids) and leukotrienes (inflammatory compounds produced when oxygen interacts with polyunsaturated fatty acids), and work with vitamin C in its antioxidant capacity. They are in large part the medicinal factor in most of the herbs sold today. If you are consuming a lot of leafy vegetables and fruits daily, you may be getting about 1 gm. per day.

In addition to the 500 mg. in LEM, my clients have reported relief from their allergies when they add 2 gm. of bioflavonoids and 4 or more gm. of vitamin C daily throughout the day at the first sign of an allergy attack and continue until the allergy is under control. The allergy sometimes comes back as the dose is lowered and then dissipates as it is increased. If that amount does not work for you, bump it up a bit until you find relief.

Twinlab makes a good bioflavonoid mixture that can be purchased through the Prolongevity company.

**Bromelain (15 mg.)** is a proteolytic enzyme found in raw pineapple that stimulates protein synthesis and repair. It slowly dissolves away damaged protein (scar tissue, etc.) and, therefore, speeds up healing rates.

Over the past twenty years, I have had tendinitis in various parts of my body because of participation in racquet sports and other body pounding activities such as running and aerobics. Tendinitis is inflammation of the tendon and/or the insertion point of tendon to muscle or tendon to bone caused by excessive pounding activities. Most doctors' advice is to take ibuprofen (or any other anti-inflammatory) for the pain and stay away from the activity that causes the pain for several months and longer. I was not, and neither have my clients been, happy with that advice. In December, 1993, I developed severe wrist tendinitis (the kind that keeps you awake at night; the worst I have had). I knew there had to be a cure. I began my research and continued finding sources stating that bromelain is an anti-inflammatory and a good digestive aid for protein. I surmised, based on all evidence discovered, that tendinitis created an internal wound resulting in scar tissue (fibrous material composed of calcium ions and protein). I then theorized that tendinitis could be cured by ingesting bromelain, but I could not find anything in the literature concerning how much to take. I became my own guinea pig for this project, too. I began with 750 mg. per day in divided doses. I did not feel significant relief until I increased the dosage to 1,500 mg. per day in divided doses. Then it took about two weeks for the pain to go away completely.

I believe the combination of anti-inflammatory action and protein dissolving abilities enables bromelain to do this job. Significant amounts of vitamins C and E, beta-carotene, bioflavonoids, and zinc, similar to those found in LEM, are necessary constituents to bromelain for it to be effective.

Bromelain has also been found to be useful in reducing the soreness of and speeding the healing of bruises, reducing pain and swelling after oral surgery, and aiding in the digestion of protein-rich foods. Papain, another protein dissolving enzyme like bromelain, is one of the main ingredients found in meat tenderizers.

## Herbal Antioxidant Complex

**Grape seed extract (20 mg.)** made by Indena contains 95 percent of the active ingredient proanthocyanidin. It protects the body from free radical damage that occurs in cells with limited blood flow, such as the blood brain barrier neurons and inflamed joint linings. It also protects against age-related degradation of the elastin under the skin, therefore helping to maintain youthful appearance. It also works along with bilberry extract to improve microcapillary circulation throughout the body.

**Bilberry extract (10 mg.)**, containing 25 percent anthocyanin made by Chemco has been shown in studies to protect against cardiovascular problems, skin problems, rheumatoid arthritis, and eye related disorders, including diabetic retinopathy.

**Milk thistle extract (20 mg.)** with 85.5 percent silymarin has been successfully used to shrink tumors and treat toxic chemical and alcohol-induced liver diseases of various kinds, including cirrhosis, chronic hepatitis, and inflammation of the bile duct.

## Vitamin B Complex

**Vitamin B1 (thiamin) (200 mg.)** is a co-factor with vitamin B6 in fighting atherosclerosis and arthritis. It is an immune system stimulant that helps to detoxify cancer causing chemicals from cigarette smoke, car exhaust, and charcoaling. It helps protects the liver and brain from acetaldehyde poisoning (an alcohol and cigarette by-product) and helps to convert blood sugar to usable energy, thus helping hypoglycemics and diabetics. It is also helpful in the treatment of anemia. About half the vitamin B1 in our bodies is in our muscles, meaning that during exercise it postpones the onset of fatigue along with the help of vitamin B6.

**Vitamin B2 (riboflavin) (50 mg.)** turns your urine bright yellow and is soon depleted in those who do strenuous aerobic activities. It possibly protects against cancer of the esophagus and is believed to help the body absorb iron. Many cases of iron deficient anemia are believed to be due in part to vitamin B2 and vitamin C deficiency, not iron deficiency. You cannot overdose on vitamin B2, but you can on iron; consequently I do not recommend iron supplementation. By order of the government, most of our foods are fortified with iron.

**Vitamin B3 (niacin) (75 mg.) and (niacinamide—the buffered kind) (100 mg.)** are included in this combination in LEM. Niacin is known mainly for its ability to lower bad cholesterol while raising good cholesterol as we consume 1,200 mg. to 2,000 mg. per day. As with any supplement, build up to these levels (see the warnings at the end of this chapter). *Niacin* also lowers triglyceride levels (blood fats). *Niacinamide* does none of the above. *Niacinamide* and *niacin* together have been found to reduce the risk of those who are prone to heart attacks and detoxifies pollutants, alcohol, and narcotics. *Niacin* is a vasodilator (expands blood vessels) that increases blood flow and causes a constant small drain of histamines, a process that is good for allergies and asthma. This small drain of histamines may cause a tingling or itching sensation if taken on an empty stomach. The sensation dissipates in about 30 to 45 minutes. Some report that sexual activity is enhanced when 200-500 mg. of niacin is taken on an empty stomach 30 to 60 minutes before sex. You are getting a total of 750 mg. each day (nine tablets) from LEM *with extra niacin. Niacin* helps some people with sleep problems. Furthermore, very large doses of niacin (9 gm. per day) have helped schizophrenic and mental retardation patients. Arthritic conditions have improved greatly with 4-5 gms. of *niacinimide* in divided doses throughout the day.

There have been recent reports that high intakes of niacin may exacerbate existing liver conditions. I, therefore, recommend LEM *without extra niacin.* If lowering your cholesterol levels is your objective, then try *extra fiber, aerobic exercise, and extra chromium.*

**Vitamin B5 (calcium pantothenate) (600 mg.)** is revered as the athlete's vitamin. It enhances endurance and stamina; increases antibody production; improves symptoms of rheumatoid arthritis, osteoarthritis, and morning stiffness; helps with the processes involving the neurotransmitter acetylcholine (essential for good mental functioning); helps to protect us from the toxic effects of all kinds of smoke; plays a role with vitamin B3 in the gradual removal (two to three years) of "age spots," which are actually rancid fats; and gently stimulates peristalsis (the movement of wastes through the large intestine; much more desirable than a commercial laxative).

**Vitamin B6 (pyridoxine) (175 mg.)** complements vitamin B12 in the communication process between nerve cells, is essential for childrens' growth and development, works together with vitamins A, C, and E in combating arthritis and rheumatism by shrinking swollen joint membranes, and dissolves rancid fat deposits. It protects and/or corrects carpal tunnel syndrome after two to three months of 100-200 mg. per day; breaks down atherosclerotic plaque; and relieves the symptoms associated with premenstrual syndrome (PMS), especially when combined with potassium (some excellent sources are bananas, potatoes, cantaloupe, and skim milk) and magnesium. It is possibly effective against monosodium glutamate (MSG) syndrome in susceptible people, boosts immune system function, helps control melanoma cancer in lab animals and humans, helps some diabetics, and remedies some problems associated with oral contraceptive consumption.

Vitamin B6 reduces the therapeutic effect of the drug levodopa, which is used to treat Parkinson's disease, yet it is okay to take vitamin B6 with the levodopa drug Sinemet.

Vitamin B6 may be toxic in doses of 2,000 mg. or more per day. Researchers have reported *reversible* nerve damage in four of seven patients who had been taking these incredible amounts for two to four months. Five of the seven were women, two of whom were advised by their gynecologists to take the excessive amounts. One of the two men was taking these amounts as advised by his psychiatrist.

**Vitamin B12 (cobalamin) (100 mcg.)** helps those who suffer from pernicious anemia; helps patients recover faster from viral and bacterial diseases and surgical procedures; improves mental functioning; protects, along with folic acid against smoke-induced cancer; and protects against toxins and allergens such as sulfites (a common food, wine, and prescription drug additive). Those of you who are allergic to sulfites may find relief by taking 2,000-4,000 mcg. (not mg.) of vitamin B12 per day. Vegetarians, who are notoriously low in vitamin B12, particularly need the 100 mcg. in LEM.

**PABA (paraaminobenzoic acid) (50 mgs.)** is a B vitamin that has no number. It is a topical sunscreen, a membrane stabilizer that protects red blood cells from bursting, protector against ozone toxicity, and can sometimes prevent hair loss and return gray hair back to its original color (maybe 10 percent of all cases).

Discontinue use if you are on any kind of sulfa drug; the combination has caused nausea and diarrhea in some individuals. Fifty mg. is a modest dose compared to those who have had problems with the ingestion of 1,000 mg. or more daily.

**Folic acid (folate triglutamate) (800 mcg.)** protects against lung and bronchial cancer (particularly those around cigarette smoke); prevents birth defects; is beneficial in the treatment of mental retardation; helps in the treatment of cervical dysplasia, an abnormality of the cervix and may precede cervical cancer; is required along with vitamin B12 to produce red blood cells in bone marrow, thus lending to the support of the necessity to prevent pernicious anemia; may help to relieve symptoms of psoriasis and gingivitis; and has been shown to be beneficial in the treatment of candida (a yeast infection that interferes with progesterone and possibly estrogen function).

**Biotin (200 mcg.)** produces healthy hair and nails, prevents graying and baldness in some, and tames cowlicks. It also works synergistically with insulin making it helpful in the treatment of diabetes. Biotin defiency has also been associated with seborrhoeic dermatitis; a skin problem

91

## VITAMIN-MINERAL ANTIOXIDANT COMPLEX

**Vitamin E (50 percent Roche synthetic or 50 percent Henkel or Eastman natural) (500 IU)** protects against neurological disorders, a precancerous condition called mammary dysplasia, heart disease, air pollution, cigarette smoke, complications associated with premature infants (preemies), and the harmful side effects of radiation and chemotherapy. It assists the mineral selenium in inhibiting breast cancer in some experimental animals. Vitamin E also helps calcium and magnesium in the process of reducing the symptoms of PMS (premenstrual syndrome), relieves leg and foot muscular cramps, is effective against intermittent claudication (decreased blood flow and pain in a particular extremity), boosts the immune system, and is an extremely effective antioxidant against the peroxidation of fatty tissues. The fat in our bodies is similar to a hunk of hamburger meat exposed to oxygen. After a period of time, the meat rots or spoils (as a result of the free radical activity associated with rancidity) and smells bad. The more fat we have, the greater possibility of developing disease due to free radical activity.

If you are on anti-coagulant drugs, do not take more than 400 I.U. of Vitamin E per day. Under normal conditions, no adverse effects have been reported with doses as high as 1,600 I.U. per day.

**Vitamin A (5,000 IU)** is very effective at anti-infection, cancer protection, and immunity enhancement. It also assists zinc in the elimination of skin disorders, such as acne and psoriasis, and prevents or reverses skin aging. It speeds the healing process of wounds, fights atherosclerosis (blockages formed on the inside of artery walls causing heart attacks), acts as an internal sunscreen, and alleviates the side effects of radiation therapy.

Vitamin A can be toxic at levels greater than 20,000 I.U. per day in some people. It is fat soluble, meaning it is possible to accumulate in tissues over a period of time if taken daily in amounts greater than 20,000 I.U. Some have reported no toxic side effects in amounts as high as 100,000 I.U. The carotenes, a form of vitamin A mentioned on page 83

92

that are not fat soluble, are used by the body only as needed, thus there are no known toxicities.

**Selenium (selenate) (50 mcg.) and (seleno-methionine) (50 mcg.)** is a mineral that used to be found abundantly in our soils until the advent of chemical fertilizers, herbicides, and pesticides. It protects against various forms of cancer. Populations in such places as Rapid City, South Dakota; Venezuela; and Japan show high levels of selenium in their soils with an associated low cancer rate. It also acts as an immune system stimulant. Low levels of selenium have been found in patients with acquired immune deficiency syndrome (AIDS). Selenium also protects against heart disease and stroke. The "stroke belt" of the U.S., parts of Georgia and the Carolina's, has very low soil selenium content and high stroke and heart attack rates, as does Finland and parts of China. Selenium also detoxifies heavy metals such as cadmium and mercury; neutralizes the free radical activity in peroxidized fats; protects against cystic fibrosis along with vitamins A and E; and helps along with vitamin E to protect against tissue damage and pain associated with angina (extreme pain associated with partial shut-off of blood and oxygen to the heart).

Do not exceed 200 mcg. (not mg.) per day. Reports of garlic odor on breath, fragile fingernails, metallic taste, and nausea have been reported at this excessive level.

**Zinc (35 mg.)** is a mineral found in many high-fat foods, giving us good reason to follow the extra 25 to 50 mg. per day dose that I recommend on page 77. Plant foods and iron interfere with zinc absorption. Most of our foods are fortified with iron, and the iron content in most commercial vitamin-mineral supplements have more iron than zinc; and as mentioned throughout the book, iron toxicity can be a problem.

For infants, human breast milk has been shown to enhance zinc absorption when compared with formula or cows milk. Zinc is associated with healthier pregnancies, helpful in the treatment of mental decline associated with cirrhosis of the liver, useful along with A in treating acne and other skin disorders, and helps in the treatment of rheumatoid arthritis. Zinc is also beneficial in the treatment of diabetes, increases sperm count and testosterone levels, enhances male potency and sex drive, accelerates wound healing, helps prevent blindness as we age, boosts the immune system, and is beneficial in the treatment of Wilson's disease.

Do not exceed 150 mg. per day. Gastrointestinal problems such as nausea, excessive gas, and colic have been reported by some.

## AMINO ACID ANTIOXIDANT COMPLEX

**L-Taurine (500 mg.)** has been shown in clinical studies to improve the conditions of congestive heart failure, inhibit lung fibrosis (a toughening or non-elastic characteristic creating shortness of breath), and lower cholesterol levels in some people. It protects against cataracts and cell free radical damage, helps vegetarians who are on an imbalanced protein intake, and is possibly effective against gall bladder disease.

Taurine is a very important amino acid in mother's milk for the newborn and is thought by some to be responsible for epilepsy if the infant is deprived. Deficiency has been shown to impair vision in the developing infant. The first part of breast milk is very watery; and as the infant keeps feeding, the fat and particularly protein with taurine in it, come along when needed.

Taurine is also associated with zinc in healthy eye functions and is possibly involved with vitamins A, C, B complex, and E in slowing the incidence of or helping with the problems of Down's syndrome and muscular dystrophy. Deficiencies of taurine occur in cancer patients undergoing radiation/chemotherapy. The amounts taken in studies related to heart, cholesterol, lung, and chemotherapy were administered at much higher levels (3-6 gm.) than the 500 mg. included in the full LEM dose. Only so much of everything can be crammed into a pill. You can take extra taurine if you are treating any of the above conditions.

**N-Acetyl-Cysteine (100 mg.)** is a free radical scavenger and protects against toxins and pollutants, including cigarette smoke and alcohol. The consumption of at least three times as much vitamin C to cysteine is needed to prevent bladder and kidney stones. It is the most abundant nutrient in human hair, comprising about eight percent. Deficiency can lead to unhealthy hair and/or hair loss and dandruff.

**L-Glutathione (15 mg.)** can turn vitamins C and E back to their fresh state if they become oxidized and works with selenium as a detoxifying agent by attaching itself to dichlorodiphenyltrichloroethane (DDT—a dangerous pesticide), chlorine, bromine, lead, cadmium, and mercury and carrying them out via the urinary system. It also helps protect the liver from damage caused by alcohol, is protective against hepatitis, is used in eye surgery to bathe the eye, and offers cancer protection.

## MINERAL COMPLEX

**Magnesium (oxide, aspartate, and succinate) (1,000 mg.).** The oxide, aspartate, and succinate forms make up 600 mg. of the 1,000 mg. listed above. That leaves 400 mg. of elemental or usable magnesium. It lowers high blood pressure, helps alleviate symptoms associated with PMS, facilitates oxygen delivery to the working muscle, is a necessary constituent with calcium in the production of adenosine triphosphate (ATP—the energy reserve of the muscle). It helps protect against cardio-vascular disease, is effective in preventing calcium oxalate stones in those who have this recurrent problem, is effective in the treatment of convulsions and premature labor in women and may have a laxative effect if taken in extremely high doses. It is lost from sweating and is dangerously low in those who use diuretics. When combined with potassium, magnesuim encourages the post working muscle to relax to avoid cramping.

Although toxicity is rare, do not exceed 600 mg. elemental per day. Many over the counter laxatives contain magnesium, and abuse can cause diarrhea.

**Calcium (citrate and stearate forms) (750 mg.)** is beneficial in the treatment or prevention of osteoporosis and arthritic related diseases. The moment there is a deficiency, the body begins taking it from our bones. Females start showing bone loss at about the age of 18 and males at about

95

age 30. It is also a colorectal cancer preventive, is better than blood pressure drugs in treating high blood pressure, is largely dependent upon vitamin D for absorption, and needs magnesium at a ratio of two parts calcium to one part magnesium.

Of the 750 mg. in LEM, only about 140 mg. are usable by the body. Calcium and other minerals need a vehicle such as citrate, stearate or other forms to deliver it to the tissues so it can be utilized in the body. Therefore, only about one-fifth of the 750 mg. in LEM is calcium.

*Extension Calcium* from Vitamin Research Products also on page 77 is one of the best mineral combinations I have found. Six capsules contain 200 I.U. of vitamin D-3, 60 mcg. of vitamin K, 2 mg. of boron, 1,000 mg. of calcium, 1 mg. of copper, 150 mg. of magnesium, 4 mg. of manganese, and 25 mg. of silicon dioxide. All the above amounts in Extension Calcium are elemental or usable amounts. Men should take six per day and women should take eight. If you are an athlete involved in body pounding/vibrating activities such as golf, running, walking, weight training, etc., then I recommend two more per gender.

Another form of tendinitis, which I had at one time, is called calcium tendinitis. It is related to mineral deficiencies. It can take several months to feel the positive effects of consuming Extension Calcium along with LEM.

If you do choose LEM as your main staple, beware of mineral combinations containing higher amounts of magnesium than Extension Calcium above. You may develop stools that are a little too soft. Diarrhea may even result.

**Potassium (99 mg.)** protects against hypertension (high blood pressure) and stroke related deaths. Studies show the relationship between sodium and potassium to be the high blood pressure culprit. Generally, where there is high sodium in populations, there is low potassium. Potassium rich foods generally cost more than sodium rich foods; thus impoverished populations have a higher incidence of stroke and high blood pressure. Scientific literature shows that if potassium is increased and sodium stays the same, blood pressure, and strokes drop. Try to attain a 2:1 ratio of potassium to sodium. The government allows only 99 mg. to be put in a daily dose where supplements are concerned. Raw fruits, vegetables, and skim milk are some of the best sources of potassium. *This is one of the very few areas where food provides more than the pill form.* It improves athletic performance in those who are deficient. Those who train 3-4 hours daily can lose up to 700 mg. from sweat, about the same amount in one banana.

Most of us typically consume 2,000-3,000 mg. of salt daily. For example: Food manufacturers transform 3.5 ounces of fresh raw peas containing 380 mg. of potassium and 2 mg. of sodium into 236 mg. of sodium, and at the same time, decrease the potassium content to 160 mg. by the canning process. The same thing applies to other common vegetables like broccoli, spinach, and Brussels sprouts. When salting your foods, if you really have to, try a salt substitute (potassium chloride).

**Vitamin D3 (cholecalciferol) (300 IU)** can be absorbed via a process initiated by the sun yet is not very abundant in the food chain, even though it is fortified in some of our foods in the U.S. Those in very northern climates, or those who get fewer than 20 minutes of sunlight per day, are prone to vitamin D deficiency. For those who use sunscreens, supplementary sources are increasingly important. It also promotes calcium and phosphorus absorption for normal bone growth, protects against cancer of the colon and breast, and is beneficial in the treatment of already acquired leukemia, breast, malignant melanoma, lymphoma, and colon cancer.

There is a possibility of hypercalcemia (high levels of blood calcium) at 1,000 IU of vitamin D. Some symptoms of hypercalcemia include nausea, drowsiness, confusion, high blood pressure, and constipation.

**Chromium (ChromeMate-niacin bound) (50 mcg.) and chromium picolinate (Nutrition 21) (50 mcg.)** is a mineral that helps your body utilize sugar. About 200 years ago, people consumed about one third of an ounce (2 teaspoons) of sugar per day. Today it is about 30 teaspoons per day or 100 pounds per year. Those of you who are diabetic or hypoglycemic have not handled this huge amount of sugar very well. The pancreas is over-burdened as it works overtime to pump insulin in an attempt to handle all that sugar.

Those of us who exercise utilize 30 teaspoons per day a lot better than those who do not. Sugar actually becomes a short term fuel for the muscle. When not used as a fuel, it turns into fat. Sugar is a simple carbohydrate, meaning it has a shorter metabolic pathway to its muscle destination than complex carbohydrates. The complex carbohydrates (mainly fruits and vegetables) are the longer lasting fuel of the two for the exercising muscle.

Chromium is very beneficial in helping diabetics and non-diabetics metabolize sugar, reduce cholesterol and triglyceride (blood fats) levels, and reduce the craving for sweets and food in general by signaling the satiety center. It is deficient mostly among the aged, pregnant women, and regular exercisers.

The typical American diet is below 50 mcg. (not mg.) per day. Studies show that we need 200-500 mcg. per day. You are getting 100 mcg. from LEM and another 200 mcg. if you are following my recommendations on page 77.

**Molybdenum (sodium molybdate) (125 mcg.)** counteracts the harmful effects of sulfites (used to preserve foods, wines, and prescription drugs) and mercury poisoning (dental fillings, etc.), and fights the negative effects of formaldehyde found in pressed-wood products, furniture, carpets, upholstery, foam insulation, paper products, and cosmetics. Formaldehyde causes the body's defense system to attack itself.

Molybdenum also protects people from esophageal cancer. The highest incidence of this form of cancer has been found in a province in North China and South Africa. The soil levels in these areas are very low in molybdenum.

**Manganese (gluconate) (5 mg.)** curbs the harmful effects of mercury; assists with zinc and chromium in helping the pancreas regulate blood sugar; helps the body process ammonia, which in high amounts can lead to diabetic coma; and is possibly useful in the treatment of osteoarthritis.

**Iodine (kelp) (10 mcg.)** deficiency is related to the formation of goiters (a golf ball-sized or larger growth on the neck). It is a sign of an underactive thyroid gland. The thyroid needs iodine to make its hormone thyroxine, which is related to the amount of energy you have. If you are tired, depressed, or physically colder than others and are having a hard time losing weight (these symptoms precede the goiter), you may need an iodine boost. If you do not use table salt, eat many seafood products, including kelp, then you may be deficient. Iodine also relieves pain and soreness associated with fibrocystic breasts and protects against radioactive poisoning.

## CHOLINERGIC COMPLEX

**Choline bitartrate (500 mg.) and phosphatidyl choline (150 mg.)** has been shown to help in memory tasks in the young and old alike. Choline is the precursor to acetylcholine, the chemical that plays a vital role in the processing, storage, and retrieval of information in the brain. The senile and those with Altzheimer's disease have been particularly helped. Vitamin B5 is required for the synthesis of acetylcholine. The studies that have been done with choline alone did not show the same positive results. Certain trycyclic anti-depressants, anti-histamines, and anti-spasmodics have been shown to counteract the positive effects of choline. It is also helpful in the treatment of tartive dyskinesia (a disorder that causes twitching and jerking movements of the facial muscles and tongue and sometimes the muscles of the trunk and extremities) and seems to work better in the treatment of manic depression than the standard therapy of lithium and other psychiatric drugs without the side effects. These studies used much greater amounts of phosphatidyl choline (15-30 gm.). Phosphatidyl choline contains about 10 percent choline. Lecithin turns into choline in the body and is helpful in the treatment of viral and non-viral (such as alcohol induced) hepatitis.

Very high daily doses of phosphatidyl choline (200 gm.) have produced the side effects of nausea, dizziness, and a fishy odor in some people.

**Inositol (250 mg.)** is a sugar found in muscles and, therefore, acts as a fuel for the working muscle. It also has a protective effect on hair follicles and brings back the natural coloring of a person's graying hair in about 10 percent of all cases and is helpful in treating a condition called diabetic peripheral neuropathy (damage to nerve fibers because of high blood pressure). The amounts taken for diabetic peripheral neuropathy were at doses of 1,000 to 1,650 mg. daily.

## SECONDARY ANTIOXIDANTS

**Dilaurylthiodipropionate (25 mg.) and thiodipropionic acid (25 mg.)** help prevent the formation of peroxides (oxidized fats), are added to foods to keep them from becoming rancid, and exhibit a very positive relationship with ascorbyl palmitate (fat-soluble vitamin C).

# CHAPTER 21

## SUPPLEMENTS FOR OTHER NEEDS
## NOT INCLUDED IN LEM

**D, L-Phenylalanine (500 mgs.)** is a common size of this 50-50 blend of the d and l forms of phenylalanine, an amino acid. D is used to relieve pain. L is used as an appetite suppressant, stimulant, and antidepressant. Phenylalanine is used by the brain to produce norepinephrine, a hormone depleted by stress and some pharmacological and recreational drugs. Since it competes with other amino acids, take it upon awakening on an empty stomach in order for it to pass through the blood brain barrier. The recommended dosage is 500-1,000 mg. If this amount produces insomnia, cut the dose in half. It should be combined with vitamins B6 and C. The amounts of B6 and C that you are getting in LEM are sufficient. Phenylalanine and caffeine make a good combination. Caffeine depletes the hormone norepinephrine, and phenylalanine replaces it. Caffeine gives us a temporary lift by using the hormone without replacing it.

Phenylalanine should be used with caution by those with hypertension, phenylketonuria (PKU, a genetic defect of the brain), or pre-existing pigmented melanoma, (a type of skin cancer) and should not be used in combination with anti-depressant drugs.

This product can be purchased from Prolongevity, Life Services Supplements, Twin Lab, and Vitamin Research Products.

**Creatine Monohydrate** is a body sculpting supplement that naturally occurs in red meat and replenishes adenosine triphosphate (ATP). ATP is the powerhouse of the muscle cell. Significant muscular growth and, hence, strength are noticed within two weeks when using this supplement as directed below. If you are trying to lower body fat, creatine indirectly helps by increasing your metabolic rate: more muscle = higher metabolic rate.

Consider the idea that your car engine is a six cylinder, and you have always driven it with five spark plugs (assume you did not know any better). It always got you from point A to point B; and you, therefore, never knew its full potential. One day your mechanic discovers the missing plug and installs it; and you are elated by the increased performance. It is now running at its full potential and getting better gas mileage.

You can give your muscles the sixth spark plug by using creatine because it facilitates muscle growth and, concurrently, strength in a very short period of time. What this process can mean to you is that you will: (1) be able to perform better athletically, (2) have a better chance of catching yourself if you fall, thus avoiding injury, (3) burn more calories at rest or during exercise because of the extra muscle mass, and (4) have an even better looking body than you now have because muscle, in the opinion of most people, is prettier than fat.

To dispel any myths, you will not: (A) turn into "Muscles McGurk" or (B) lose body fat if your caloric intake exceeds your expenditure.

Those of us who have been training with weights for years (not the body building regimen), reach a plateau and stay there. My routine in the weight room for the past five years has remained consistently the same. It involves six sets of four to six repetitions. I kept the same routine during the testing phase while taking this supplement.

I started taking creatine on November 21, 1994. After two weeks, my weight went from 146 pounds to 152 pounds. My body fat percentage stayed the same at 8.3 percent. Four weeks after first taking it, my weight went up two more pounds to 154, *equating to eight pounds of muscle in approximately one month.* My body fat remained at 8.3 percent. If you are heavier than I, you will most likely experience greater gain. If you are lighter, you most likely will experience less gain. The amount of weight that I work out with went up 20 percent from November 21, 1994 to December 17, 1994. That is significant for anyone, athlete or not.

Creatine continually replenishes ATP. It keeps the muscle contracting effectively and efficiently. The exercising muscle continually uses creatine at a fast rate; much faster than the sedentary muscle. You would have to eat five to six pounds of beef per day to get the amount the supplemental form provides, thus explaining why our muscles will grow if we keep our creatine stores up. Creatine is one of the forty plus supplements our foods are not supplying in adequate amounts. Another bonus of supplementation is that it combines with phosphorus to help buffer lactic acid buildup. *Lactic acid is the waste product of exercise that enhances fatigue and muscular soreness.*

One study examined the effects of creatine on a muscular degenerative eye disease called gyrate atrophy of the choroid and retina, which can lead to blindness. Creatine halted the progression of the disease, and the subjects gained ten percent in lean body mass without exercise. My point in bringing up this particular study is that it may be possible for you to increase your lean mass without exercise just by taking creatine. I, of course, do not advise abstaining from exercise; but this information may be helpful to those who have muscular degenerative diseases that prevent them from exercising.

**There are two phases involved in taking creatine.**
**The loading and the maintenance phase is as follows:**

**Loading phase**: *The first five days* mix one heaping teaspoon (approximately five grams) in your favorite beverage or water four times per day for a total of twenty grams.

**Maintenance phase**: After completing the loading phase, take one heaping teaspoon per day thirty minutes to an hour before exercise "until the end of time."

Creatine can become *creatinine* if left in liquid for fifteen minutes or more. *Creatinine* is the by-product of creatine and is found in blood tests as a measure of how much creatine we have in our muscles. Consume it immediately after you mix it up or just eat it dry. It has no taste.

Muscle atrophy (degeneration) occurs when a muscle is not exercised as you have probably seen when someone has a broken limb in a cast for a period of time. If you discontinue using creatine, your muscles will decrease to their original size prior to taking it, even if you continue to lift weights. If you stop taking creatine and stop exercising, then you will notice muscle atrophy even more.

*This is not a steroid!* It does not put on synthetic muscle nor does it have any side effects.

This product can be purchased from Vitamin Research Products.

**Ornithine Alpha-Ketoglutarate (OKG)** is an amino acid combination that facilitates the release of growth hormone via the pituitary gland. Growth hormone production declines dramatically as we approach our thirties. Eating high fat foods and not exercising large muscle groups contributes to the decline of growth hormone in all ages. Having growth hormone circulating in our bodies helps us metabolize fat, build muscle (anabolic), increase bone strength, thicken our skin to youthful levels, and heal in about half the time compared to those who have depressed levels. Some studies have shown remarkable results in muscle growth and reductions in body fat in highly trained young athletes. New studies done on burn patients and on patients undergoing surgery show clearly that OKG maintains muscle during severe trauma. Injuries generally cause significant muscle loss (catabolism).

OKG works best when taken on an *empty stomach before bedtime and/or before exercise*. Avoid taking OKG with supplements containing other amino acids such as protein and LEM. It is more effective when it does not have to compete with other amino acids. Schedule OKG consumption at least two hours away from your other supplements and/or food.

This product can be purchased from Vitamin Research Products.

**Protein** supplementation, contrary to common beliefs shared by many college and university colleagues, is of great benefit to all exercisers. The research backing the benefits can no longer be ignored. I use it and am pleased with the results. Muscular gains are slower than that when using creatine; yet I am happy with my personal findings.

The physiological principles of protein supplementation are simple: *Exercise grows muscle, period.* Protein supplementation provides a positive environment for the muscle to grow. *Protein supplementation without exercise will not produce muscle growth.* Supplementation provides a positive nitrogen balance in the body. Negative nitrogen balance puts the body in a catabolic state (muscle cannibalism), the state that most exercisers are in when they do not use protein supplement correctly. The amino acids (protein) in the right amounts are necessary for the anabolic state (muscle growth) or for maintaining the amount of muscle you now have. As we age, we lose muscle on a slow, consistent basis if we do not take the steps necessary to prevent the loss. If you recall, muscle is metabolically active; and the slow loss of muscle contributes to our fat stores.

Vegetarian diets are notoriously low in protein. They contain protein but in the wrong ratios to maintain a positive nitrogen balance. Generally, consuming food *without* protein supplementation *will not* provide the positive environment needed to grow muscle and will not keep you from losing muscle if you exercise aerobically (activities that require oxygen) or anaerobically (activities that do not require oxygen). There is an exception to the above statement: if you consume mass quantities of egg whites or other high protein foods regularly you may stay in a positive nitrogen balance but the biological value of food protein is not as good as the protein supplement recommended on page 109.

Aerobic activities make your body need extra protein because you are creating a negative nitrogen balance. Have you ever noticed distance runners with well developed butt, thighs, and calves but *comparatively* very small upper bodies? If you deplete your muscles of glycogen (fuel formed from carbohydrates), the body literally eats its own muscle (mainly upper body in this case) for fuel. Losses of protein in sweat, respiration, and hemolysis (death of red blood cells) increase dramatically as you exercise.

Burn patients and those with other traumas display severe muscle loss. Their protein requirements are as high as athletes in intense training. People in this desperate state have suppressed immune systems, and the proper protein intake enhances the immune system.

Studies prior to 1974 used sedentary individuals confined to metabolic wards as subjects for protein studies; and, therefore, most colleagues whom I mentioned before "hang their hats" on the Recommended Daily Allowances (RDAs). The RDA equates to approximately **.36** grams of protein per pound of bodyweight. Uninformed professors, physicians, nutritionists, and dieticians who are funded by the meat and dairy industries still encourage you to eat their high fat products for protein fulfillment. If the proteins that you eat are inadequate or inferior, the structures of your body will be inadequate and inferior. Because of the RDA's being set at such a low range, it is easy for us to reach the **.36** grams per pound of body weight by consuming the high fat meat and dairy products.

Dr. I. Gontzea and colleagues at the Institute of Medicine in Bucharest were the first to show in 1974 that exercising bodies need more than the RDA. For two weeks they gave sedentary athletes (not in training at the time of the study) **.48** grams of protein per pound of body weight. That amount is 72 grams for a 150-pound person, equating to 33 percent more than the RDA. They stayed in a positive nitrogen balance. After the two-week sedentary period, they instructed the athletes to workout for two hours per day. Nitrogen balance dropped to negative within two days. So protein intake one third higher than the RDA put them into the *catabolic* state when they exercised two hours a day.

Dr. Gontzea then fed protein to another group of athletes in amounts twice the RDA of **.72** grams per pound of body weight, which is 108 grams for a 150-pound person. As long as they remained sedentary, their nitrogen balance stayed positive. When they began exercising for two hours a day, it took four days for their nitrogen balance to drop to the negative status.

A study conducted at Tufts University by Dr. William Evans and colleagues showed that men who exercise regularly and moderately (less than two hours/day) in endurance sports such as swimming, running, and/or cycling need about **.64** grams of protein per pound of body weight on days of exercise, equating to 96 grams for a 150-pound person.

Dr. Peter Lemon, a leading researcher in the area of protein, found that endurance athletes need 25-50 percent more protein than the RDA, dependent on the intensity and duration of the activity.

A study reported in *The Physician and Sports Medicine* showed that weight trainers (those who spend lots of time in the gym) need protein at a rate of 438 percent higher than the RDA to keep them in a positive nitrogen balance, equating to about two grams per pound of body weight; 300 grams for a 150-pound person.

I discovered that I need 85-160 grams per day (including the amount in my food) to grow muscle, depending upon how much activity I have per day. During my testing period (January 14-August 30, 1995), my weight went from 154 to 158 with body fat level at 8.3 percent equating to about one half pound per month. My lifting days were only two per week, one hour each, and I would do a full body workout each time for a total of two hours per week (compared to some lifters, not a lot of time with weights). My aerobic activities would consist of one to two hours five to six days per week. On the days that I lifted and did aerobic activities, I consumed the high range of 160 grams. From August 31, 1995 to November 4, 1995, I stopped protein consumption completely except for the amount in my food (about 60 grams per day). My weight slowly dropped to 151 pounds. I lost one percent in body fat, so I lost about five pounds of muscle during the two-month period.

Dr. Michael Colgan at The Colgan Institute in California created a guide for us to follow for protein supplementation. It is based on activity levels and body weight shown in the following chart (Table 21-1).

Dr. Colgan defines *Class 1* sports as those that demand strength first, then speed, then endurance. Class 1 includes weight training, shot put, javelin, discus, and men's gymnastics. *Class 2* sports are those that demand speed first, then strength, then endurance. Sprints of all kinds, jumping, boxing, wrestling, karate, judo, women's gymnastics, and most ball games are in this class. *Class 3* sports are those in which endurance dominates. These include middle and long distance running, triathlons, cross-country skiing, cycling, racquetball, and tennis.

**Table 21-1**

### DAILY PROTEIN REQUIREMENTS FOR ATHLETES
### (IN GRAMS)

| Body Weight/Pounds | Sports Training Category | | |
| --- | --- | --- | --- |
| | Class 1 | Class 2 | Class 3 |
| 88 | 80 | 68 | 56 |
| 110 | 100 | 85 | 70 |
| 132 | 120 | 102 | 84 |
| 154 | 140 | 119 | 98 |
| 176 | 160 | 136 | 112 |
| 198 | 180 | 153 | 126 |
| 220 | 200 | 170 | 140 |
| 242 | 220 | 187 | 154 |
| 264 | 240 | 204 | 168 |

Table 21-1 above is taken from *Optimum Sports Nutrition*, pg. 151: Used by permission from Advanced Research Press and The Colgan Institute.

based on maximum training levels of three hours per day or more. He says that if you put in only one to two hours per day, you need less protein and, therefore, need to move one class to the right. If you are already in Class 3, then move to the next lower bodyweight.

Dr. Colgan continues to say that the most amount of muscle gain they have measured in a year is 18.25 pounds in drug-free athletes. Based on his research, he disagrees with the magazine ads claiming "25 pounds of solid muscle in 12 weeks."

# WHICH PROTEIN IS BEST?

Egg whites, turkey, chicken, beef, etc. have low biological values (BV) compared to the protein supplement below called Designer Protein. Cooking causes cross-linking, which is an oxidation reaction causing an undesirable bond between nucleic acids and proteins (free radical activity). In this process, you get protein from foods, but it is damaged protein.

Well-processed whey hydrolysate (pre-digested) is by far the best protein on the market. It has the highest BV of any protein. BV is the measure that scientists use to rate how well nitrogen is absorbed into muscles. Studies show that whey hydrolysate is much more effective than free form amino acids, soy, egg whites, and casein proteins.

Whey contains all of the essential and nonessential amino acids and has the three branched chain amino acids (BCAAs) in the highest concentrations found in nature. The BCAAs make up one third of muscle protein. 1-Leucine, 1-Valine, and 1-Isoleucine make up the BCAAs. L-Leucine is used up faster than 1-Valine or 1-Isoleucine and, therefore, should make up the highest content of the three in the protein supplement that you choose. Space your protein consumption throughout the day. Some people have a hard time digesting more than 30 grams of protein per sitting.

If you are not taking in enough protein, you will know by watching your bodyweight and circumferential measurements drop without a drop in body fat. If you are getting too much, you will know because of a lot of low back pain and feelings of malaise. If you do not want to experience this discomfort, have a blood test for urea—called blood urea nitrogen (BUN)—during the time you are taking protein. Some labs call it Urea Nitr for short or Urea Nitrogen. The normal range varies from lab to lab. Some say 4-24 milligrams per deciliter (mg./dl.) and others say 7-25 mg./dl. Dr. Richard Passwater suggests that a BUN over 21 mg./dl. indicates poor health. My BUN measured 15 mg./dl. on July 22, 1995 while in the midst of consuming 85-160 grams of protein per day. I never experienced low back pain or feelings of malaise. If these symptoms happen to you, lower your protein consumption. After a while, you will excrete the excess and perk back up nicely.

High BUN can also be caused by dehydration. If you are not urinating every three hours, I suggest you increase your water consumption until you do.

Beware of many of the protein supplements on the market. Many contain dangerous levels of iron. Others have higher-than-needed ratios of carbohydrate to protein, meaning you would have to consume a lot of carbohydrates to get your needed protein and giving you many unnecessary calories. I would rather get my carbohydrate calories from my food.

The best protein supplement that I have found is called Designer Protein. You can get it just about anywhere. Many health food stores and pro shops carry it. Prolongevity also sells it.

**Anti-Alcohol Antioxidants** have several benefits. In one interesting study, researchers reported that a group of rats were given a dose of acetaldehyde (a poison formed as a by-product of alcohol and tobacco smoke....stuff that causes hangovers) large enough to kill 90 percent of them. A different group was given a combination of vitamin C, cysteine, and vitamin B1; and there were no deaths. Because of this study, we now know how *the right combinations of vitamin B1, vitamin C, cysteine, and glutathione* inhibit the free radical pathologies of acetaldehyde poisoning. Since alcohol is extremely dehydrating, I suggest you drink a glass of water along with each cocktail. Dehydration significantly adds to headache hangovers. An interesting side effect of taking this supplement on a regular basis is the production of stronger finger nails and thicker hair.

One capsule per drink consumed is recommended. If you happen to be taking this supplement for hair and nails, I recommend one to two capsules three times per day.

Prolongevity and Vitamin Research Products carry this product.

**Cranex Cranberry** protects against or cures urinary tract infections. The capsules are filled with a concentrated extract that is extraordinarily high in the glycoprotein inhibitor that keeps bacteria from clinging to human tissue. Two capsules contain the equivalent biological activity of 96 ounces of cranberry juice, making the pill form a much better alternative. Your fluid intake should come from water. I have had success taking two capsules every five to six hours along with my regular supplement routine. My symptoms went away after a few days, but I continued to take it for two weeks to make sure the bacteria was gone for good.

This product or one similar to it can be purchased from Prolongevity or your health food store.

**Kyolic Garlic** is a brand of garlic that is odorless and is organically grown in compost rich soil. It is the better and cheaper alternative to antibiotics, and it has numerous benefits. It lowers total cholesterol, blood pressure, and triglycerides while raising HDL cholesterol (the good one). It is effective in the treatment of yeast infections, sore throats, bladder infections, urinary tract infections, and vaginitis (*antifungal, antibacterial, and antiviral*). There is also substantial evidence that garlic is an anti-cancer agent. Recent research has shown that it can arrest as many as *sixty* fungi, including candida albicans and *twenty* types of the worst bacteria, including cryptococcal meningitis, streptococcus, and staphylococcus. Allicin and ajoene are two of the active ingredients believed to be responsible for garlics curative properties.

Many of my clients and I have succeeded in terminating various conditions such as strep throat and parasites with this brand of garlic. Each capsule contains 200 mgs. Two capsules every five to six hours are recommended for at least a two week period. Symptoms may go away after a few days, but keep taking it for two-weeks or longer, or the condition you are treating may return.

This product can be purchased from Prolongevity or health food stores.

**Flaxseed Oil—EPA/DHA** contains two essential fatty acids that we get very little of in our diets unless we consume cold water fish or take flaxseed oil on a regular basis. Studies have shown if we consume these fatty acids in the right amounts on a regular basis, we can successfully

111

treat eczema, psoriasis, lower LDL cholesterol (the bad one), elevate HDL cholesterol (the good one), decrease platelet stickiness (sticky platelets can lead to heart disease), protect against hypertension, help prevent/treat cancer (including breast cancer), relieve depression, and treat arthritis and other inflammatory diseases.

For a long time, scientists did not understand why Greenland Eskimos and coastal Japanese, who consume high amounts of fat and cold water fish, had low levels of triglycerides, cholesterol, and heart disease. Eating cold water fish held the key to this paradox. We Westerners consume many harmful fats and small amounts of cold water fish and/or flaxseed oil. We correspondingly have high rates of heart disease, depression, etc. Cold water fish and flaxseed oil are high in eicosopentaenoic (EPA) and decosahexaenoic (DHA) fatty acids. These are also called omega three (EPA) and omega six (DHA) oils. The ratio of EPA to DHA should be at least 3:1 in favor of EPA. Buy cold processed oil or capsules of either the fish oil or flaxseed oil. Fish oil can leave a fishy after taste, so you may prefer the flaxseed oil.

The recommended dosage of the straight oil is one half to one tablespoon per day in divided doses or all at once. The recommended number of capsules is three to six per day in divided doses or all at once.

Those who hemorrhage or bleed easily, as well as diabetics, should consult a competent health professional before taking this supplement. Some research groups have reported increases in blood sugar and sharp declines in insulin secretion in diabetics of both the type I and II category.

Omega Nutrition and Spectrum Naturals make a good flaxseed oil mixture. You can purchase it from L&H Vitamins or a health food store, but *do not buy it if is not in the refrigerated section.*

**Nasturtium Restorative Moisturizing Cream** is one of the best skin creams I have found. It contains modified fruit acids, which have excellent exfoliative (slough off dead skin cells) properties. It also contains many herbs known to enhance circulation in the skin, gets rid of fine wrinkles, and does not have an oily feel. This cream contains natural progesterone, another ingredient shown to have anti-aging properties

including fine line removal and skin firmness.
This product can be purchased from Prolongevity.

**Rejuvenex** is a skin cream formulated by Carmen Fusco, M.S., R.N. and is also one of my favorites. It contains several ingredients that give you younger-looking, softer skin. The ingredient, sodium pyrrolidone carboxylic acid (PCA), is a natural constituent of skin cells that attracts moisture to our skin, keeping it soft and supple. Oils do not correct the loss of sodium PCA. As we age, our skin cells lose significant amounts of sodium PCA, creating the need to replace it with creams such as this one.
This product can be purchased from Prolongevity.

**N-Zime Caps** is an enzyme preparation that aids in the digestion of carbohydrates, proteins and fat. Each capsule contains 131 mg. of amylase (for carbohydrate), 131 mg. of protease (for protein), and 15 mg. of lipase (for fat). As we age, we lose the ability to digest some foods. Signs of incomplete digestion may be excessive gas and bloating. Food allergies may also develop as a result of decreased enzyme activity.
This product can be purchased from Prolongevity.

**BioPro** introduces beneficial intestinal bacteria necessary for an efficient and effective digestive tract. Excessive gas, bloating, and diarrhea are signs these bacertia may need to be replaced. This product contains the DDS-1 strain of acidophilus, bifidum, longum, faecium, and sporogenes. There are a minimum of one billion active bacteria in every dose. A carbohydrate called fructooligosaccharides (FOS) found in foods such as bananas, tomatoes, onions, and garlic is needed by the bacteria to do their job. Antibiotics and chlorine kill bacteria indiscriminately, including beneficial bacteria. The next time you go to Mexico you might try a combination of this supplement and Kyolic Garlic instead of the antibiotic Bactrim.
This product can purchased from Vitamin Research Products in powder or capsule form.

# CHAPTER 22

## KEEP 'EM COLD

Store *all* of your supplements in the refrigerator. Most of them lose a significant amount of potency if subjected to heat and light. They have to be kept in a cool, dark place to keep them from degrading over time This explains why quality supplements come in smoke colored plastic or opaque white bottles. Vitamin C in particular can turn into a compound called dehydroascorbic acid, a strong oxidizing agent that enhances free radical activity in the body rather than stopping it. Vitamin C squelches free radical activity. Most experts recommend the storage temperature not to exceed 86 degrees Fahrenheit.

## SIDE EFFECTS

Anything consumed in amounts greater than the body is able to process in a given period of time can cause problems. We can overdose on anything. Drinking ten gallons of water per day would eventually cause the kidneys to shut down. I do not recommend, therefore, that you consume water in such quantities. I also recommend that you do not exceed the amounts of each supplement listed in this book without the consent of a *competent* health professional. There are some *reversible* side effects of a few of the listed supplements when taken in prohibitively large amounts as noted at the end of the listings for vitamins A, B3, B6, C, PABA, D3, E, and the supplement choline. The minerals magnesium, selenium, and zinc also show side effects when taken in higher doses than that listed in this book. Vitamins A, D, and E are fat soluble, meaning they can accumulate in fatty tissues over a period of time if taken in large amounts. Vitamin K is also fat soluble, but it is not included in LEM because it is one of the few supplements besides potassium that is present in sufficient amounts in the food chain. Sixty mcg. of vitamin K are contained in six capsules of Extension Calcium, a very safe level of consumption. Dangerous levels of vitamin K consumption are known at the 500 mcg. per day amount.

## POISONOUS SUPPLEMENTS

Most commercial supplements that come from pharmacies, grocery, and health food stores are food grade. Food grade contains questionable raw materials that can have as many as *40 contaminants*. Most manufacturers use food grade because of cost. They then turn around and charge you two to three times the amount that you can buy the same pharmaceutical grade for.

Have people ever told you they cannot take supplements because they are allergic to them? Like most people, they probably bought the food grade junk. Health food stores have some good products such as Twin Lab and Omega Nutrition, but they also carry a variety of undesirable products. Ingredients like tree sap, coal tars, shellac, sand, and talc are common stretchers, fillers, and binders. They may be called "inert substances" or "excipients." Animal and polyunsaturated fats are other ingredients often found in supplements. Just like the fat in your body, these fats can become rancid if they have not been refrigerated, have been exposed to too much light, have been sitting on the store shelf too long, and/or have been heat treated, a process some manufacturers use to get the pills through the filling machinery at a rapid rate.

Another big problem with the large commercially advertised and some multi-level brands is the amount of "good stuff" versus the "bad stuff" they put in their multi-formulas. Take a look at the amount of vitamin C per pill of any multi-formula that you pull off your pharmacy or grocery shelf. They typically have 60 to 90 mg. per pill. Your body needs, according to the scientific evidence, about 7,000 times that amount or more. The same goes for most all the other vitamins, minerals, and amino acids. The prohibitive amount of iron (eighteen mg. is common) many manufacturers include in their multi-formulas makes many of us sick to our stomachs. As we continue to take in this amount daily, it builds up and is unquestionably linked to heart disease and cancer of the colon, lung, bladder and esophagus. The government requires food companies to put iron in processed foods. We do need iron but not the amounts we have been oversold on. Eighteen mg. per day for pregnant women, fifteen mg. per day for non-pregnant, and ten mg. per day for men and children are the maximums we should be consuming. If you are diagnosed with iron deficient anemia, there is a good probability you are low on vitamins C and B2, which are believed to enhance iron absorption. The sad part of this scenario is that you are then advised by your doctor to increase your iron intake, creating dangerous levels.

# CHAPTER 23

## FREE RADICALS

In 1956, Dr. Denham Harman of The University of Nebraska developed the free radical theory of aging. Think of free radicals as the children who are raised with constant negative reinforcement. As they grow up, they are always in trouble: vandalism, destructive behavior, theft, and eventually criminal activities. The free radicals that Dr. Harman is talking about are oxygen molecules that cannot find a mate and destroy anything in their path. Rusting metal and rotting fruit are examples of the free radical activity that goes on outside of our bodies. Heart disease, cancer, and arthritis are examples of the destruction that goes on inside of us.

**Free radicals are responsible for most diseases known to man.** You do not feel the damage that is taking place inside of you until the disease or virus has a stranglehold on you. Then it may be too late. Your body fat percentage contributes to the rate at which the disease or virus affects you. Those with high body fat percentages have a much higher incidence of illness. We have known for decades how to stop free radical activity. Unfortunately, since the pharmaceutical industry cannot patent or make money on that knowledge, it has been suppressed. Keeping you ill keeps drug companies rich.

SMART EATS, SMART SUPPLEMENTS, AND SMART EXERCISE

## ANTIOXIDANTS = FREE RADICAL SCAVENGERS

Many VMAAEHs are antioxidants. The ones that are not have other jobs that directly or indirectly help the antioxidants. They are all synergistic, meaning they do a much better job when they have each other than when they are taken alone.

Besides being free radical scavengers, antioxidants give a tremendous boost to the immune system. Many prescription drugs are immunosuppressive. A strong immune system gives your body a much better chance of fighting disease.

## STRAIGHT FROM THE HORSE'S MOUTH

Supplementing VMAAEHs in the correct manner is virtually unknown unless you follow other authorities or the recommendations in this book.

Unfortunately, we tend to be educated by the popular media, multilevel companies, or health food store employees. It has been my experience that the individuals in these institutions know enough about VMAAEHs "to make them dangerous." They are far from being experts in this field. Of the hundreds of multi-level and health food store owners/employees with whom I have spoken, few have any idea how much VMAAEHs to take and how often to take them. Multi-level supplement related companies in particular are full of pseudo-scientific individuals. In turn, the consumer is counseled about health matters from questionable sources and ends up paying high prices for a product that can be obtained for much less from any one of the mail order companies mentioned. And, the technical support from mail order companies is unequalled.

# CHAPTER 24

## OTHER REASONS TO SUPPLEMENT VMAAEHS

• Cooking destroys significant amounts of VMAAEHs.

• Fertilizer use depletes crop soils of valuable minerals while replacing mainly three minerals: nitrogen, phosphorus, and potassium (NPK).

• Pesticides, herbicides, and fungicides are petroleum-based products known to cause many common psychological and neurological problems. They also create free radical activity and lower the amount of VMAAEHs in our foods.

• Food processing, refining, and storage destroys significant amounts of VMAAEHs.

• Environmental pollutants create free radicals, destroying significant amounts of VMAAEHs.

• Smoking and drinking create free radicals, destroying significant amounts of VMAAEHs.

• Most prescription drugs are immunosuppressive. VMAAEHs strengthen the immune system.

• Antibiotics kill harmful *and* beneficial bacteria. We need beneficial bacteria. Garlic, in my opinion, is a wiser choice than antibiotics.

• Between 150,000 and 300,000 deaths per year are attributed to doctor related (iatrogenic) disease compared to five associated with excessive VMAAEHs. Illegal drugs kill approximately 30,000 people, alcohol 100,000 people, and cigarette smoking 400,000 people yearly. While we were trying to kill each other in the Vietnam war, only 5,600 people per year died as a result.

• Approximately 800,000 American school children are prescribed a cheap form of speed each year called Ritalin, when in reality, their condition is related to nutritional deficiencies. Many researchers claim "Ritalin creates drug addicts."

• VMAAEHs are the safer, less expensive alternative to prescription drugs and surgery.

• VMAAEHs actually heal. Drugs and surgery, at best, provide temporary solutions.

## REASONS TO TAKE PRESCRIPTION DRUGS AND/OR HAVE SURGERY

• Most of the expense of prescription drugs and/or surgery is covered by insurance.

# Section III

# *Smart Exercise*

# CHAPTER 25

## SMART EXERCISE

The benefits of smart exercise are many. New and old studies alike consistently reinforce the advantages of a smart exercise program. Generally the results of these studies show regular lifelong exercise increases life expectancy. Most of us who exercise on a regular basis report feeling better, enjoying life more, and performing better at work and play. Extreme variations in exercise habits as well as failure to exercise responsibly, however, may increase mortality.

**Aerobic** activities performed a minimum of three days per week lower triglyceride (blood fats) levels, raise good cholesterol, lower bad cholesterol, lower elevated blood pressure, help to lower body fat levels along with "smart eats and smart supplements," lower the probability of contracting or dying from cancer and heart related diseases, and increase your chance of survival if you have to flee from danger.

**Aerobic** exercisers need more free radical scavengers such as vitamin C (see page 84) because of the higher than normal consumption of oxygen. I periodically encounter aerobic exercisers who are in the same shape as I once was (arthritis, bunions, stress fractures, muscle pulls or strains, etc.) because they do not take or refuse to believe that supplementing will solve their problems. A common practice in orthodox medicine is to prescribe pain killers to those who have arthritis of the hip. The patient then feels great and continues to exercise only to wear the joint to a nub and eventually may have to have hip replacement surgery. Did the doctor cure the patient's arthritis problem? If our good doctors would recommend the mineral protocol on page 77, hip replacement surgery and any of the other approximately 150 related arthritis disorders would be "diseases of the past."

**Anaerobic** activities, particularly weight training combined with smart supplements make your tendons, ligaments, bones, and muscles stronger. As a result, you will perform better athletically, catch yourself if you fall so you will not break bones (a major problem especially among the elderly), and be more attractive, thus raising your self confidence.

The two forms of exercise that make up the smart exercise routine as mentioned above are: **Aerobic**, meaning exercises that utilize the oxygen chemical system in your body, and **anaerobic**, meaning exercises that do not utilize the oxygen chemical system. Aerobic exercises are heart, lung, and vascular (blood vessel system) healthy activities. They include, but are not limited to; walking, jogging, stair climbing, rowing, aerobic dancing, and jumping rope. Activities that make the large muscle groups of your body (legs and buttocks) move *in a consistent and repetitive* fashion are considered **aerobic.** The result of this *consistent and repetitive* action causes the heart rate to elevate into the training or fat burning zone (see page 130) and keeps it there for a minimum of ten minutes. You will eventually build up the amount of time you spend on your aerobic activity(s), depending on how many calories you want to burn for the day and/or week. The chart on page 149 shows different activities that burn differing numbers of calories per hour. So, if you spend twenty minutes on an activity, you will have to divide the number of calories for the activity by three.

There are many **anaerobic** activities also. They are not considered as beneficial to the heart, lung, and vascular system as **aerobic** activities. You may think of them as "stop and go" activities. They cause your heart rate to rise into or over your zone and, as quickly, during the stop or rest cycle, lower your heart rate to the bottom of, or below, your zone. They include, but are not limited to, weight training, tennis, volleyball, softball, baseball, and interval training. They are all good activities because they burn calories over and above your BMR that you read about on page 42. The **anaerobic** activity that I encourage you to do more of than any other is weight training and/or any other progressive resistance (muscle building) exercise. Remember, the more muscle on your frame, the higher your metabolic rate is every day, twenty-four hours a day. You do not have to become a body builder or power lifter to train with weights. The weight training exercises that you are about to read about are ergonomic and time efficient.

# WHAT TIME OF DAY SHOULD I WORKOUT?

Are you a morning person or a night person? You may hear from some people that morning is the best time. Some say that afternoon or evening is best. I agree with the afternoon and evening group primarily because I am a night person. Morning exercise does not set well with me. I cherish early morning sleep. The bottom line is calories in and calories out. Most distance running events and cycle ride organizers schedule their functions in the early morning. These events are a lot of fun. They would be *more fun* if scheduled later in the day or at night (just my opinion, of course). There are some functions scheduled in the afternoon and night, just not many. You do not have to be "fast" to participate.

# AEROBIC/CARDIOVASCULAR EXERCISE

Let us first consider aerobic or cardiovascular activities. The bottom line is to get your heart rate in your training and/or fat burning zone (page 130) and keep it there for at least ten minutes. Eventually, as you get in better shape, you will be able to sustain the activity for twenty, thirty, or sixty minutes. Those of you who have never exercised aerobically or have been away from exercise for a month or more should get a medical clearance from a *competent* medical professional.

*Smart exercise* means to build up slowly. As a result, you will avoid muscular and joint soreness. Muscular and joint soreness is one of the main reasons people stop exercising or never start in the first place.

In general, many people are "turned-off" to physical activities because they have been coaxed to "jump into it full speed" or were administered the "no-pain, no-gain" philosophy. I still hear these foolish comments from supposed fitness experts, public school educators, or college fitness educators on a regular basis. *It is also very common to see these same people use a fitness related activity as punishment or a manipulative tool ("give me five laps for talking in line," etc.).* It is no wonder the majority of Americans do not exercise.

## CHECK YOUR PULSE

To get your heart rate into the zone means you will have to count how many times your heart beats in one minute. Place your middle and ring finger of either hand next to your esophagus and gently press until you feel your pulse via your carotid artery as shown in the picture at right.

The carotid artery is the passageway that sup-

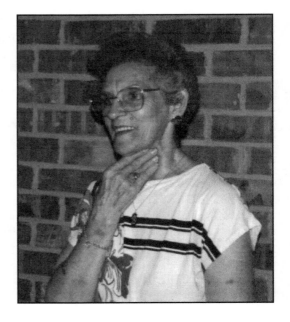

128

plies blood to your brain. You may have to pause momentarily from your exercise to check it. There are several ways to do it. The first and most accurate way is to count each beat of your heart for a full minute. Another method (a little less accurate) is to count each beat of your heart for thirty seconds and then multiply that number times two. Still another (even less accurate) is to count each beat of your heart for fifteen seconds and multiply that number times four. The quickest and least accurate way is to count each beat of your heart for six seconds and multiply that number times ten. I use the last method. For me, as many years as I have been exercising, expediency outweighs accuracy. I very seldom check mine because I know what it feels like to be in my zone. Being in your zone will be comfortable for you. You will be able to carry on a conversation with your friends as you exercise. If you get to the point of not being able to converse and are panting, huffing, and puffing, you are probably above your zone. Distance runners, swimmers, etc. are almost always above their zone when competing. On the other hand, make sure the exercise is not too easy or you will not get your heart rate up enough. Another way to monitor your heart rate is to purchase a heart rate monitor. They cost around $100 and can be purchased at any sporting goods store or from a mail order catalogue.

Table 25-1 on the following page shows how you ascertain your zone. It applies only to **aerobic**-related activities. Heart rate is not taken into consideration when you do **anaerobic** activities unless you just want to watch it erratically rise above and fall below the zone.

The most important thing to remember about exercise for burning fat is duration, not intensity. If you are not able to carry on a conversation while exercising, you are probably above your fat burning zone. Not only will you become "burned-out" and discouraged but your muscles are literally running out of gas (muscle glycogen is a by-product of carbohydrates, the main food source you are consuming with my eating plan). It is called your personal fat burning zone, even though carbohydrates are the main fuel source. You are just shifting the ratio a little more toward the fat fuel tank.

If you are not consuming a lot of fat, your body will use the fat fuel from your own fat fuel tank (thighs, gut, arms, face, etc.) instead of your

**Table 25-1**

## YOUR TRAINING AND/OR FAT BURNING ZONE

| Constant | 220 | |
|---|---|---|
| **Your Age** | | |
| Subtract age from constant which creates your estimated maximum heart rate | | |
| Your resting heart rate as you are lying down when you first awake | | |
| Subtract resting heart rate from estimated maximum heart rate | | |
| **Multiply by** | **60%** | **70%** |
| **Equals** | | |
| **Add back your resting heart rate** | | |
| **Equals your training and/or fat burning zone** | | |

glycogen fuel tank (muscles). Table 25-2 illustrates the different fuel systems utilized when exercising.

I can personally attest to the success of the "high-fat, dumb exercise"

**Table 25-2**

| Exercise | Glycogen Fuel Tank | Fat Fuel Tank |
|---|---|---|
| **1 hour above fat burning zone** | **Uses 7/8 of a tank** | **Uses 1/8 of a tank** |
| **1 hour in fat burning zone** | **Uses 1/2 of a tank** | **Uses 1/2 of a tank** |

routine. For years, I was consuming the typical high fat fare (thirty-five to forty-five percent of total calories from fat) and exercising on a very consistent basis (out of my fat burning zone though). Cycling for one to two hours every other day was not unusual. On the in-between days, I would be doing an aerobic activity such as racquetball or running. My body fat was about fifteen percent. I could not understand why I was not losing body fat with all of this activity. As time went on, I decided to get smart and started exercising with less intensity. I lowered my percentage of calories from fat to the ten to twenty percent range. I lost the protruding gut and reduced my body fat to six percent at the same time.

# DO IT CHEAP

There are many ways to get your heart rate in the zone without having to spend a lot of money on exercise equipment. As you get in shape, you may want to try a combination of ten minutes of jumping rope, ten minutes of jogging in place, and ten minutes of jumping jacks mixed with half knee bends. By mixing up different exercises with the same large muscle groups (legs and buttocks), you will be able to keep your heart rate in your zone while watching television or listening to your favorite music without getting bored. Some people have the ability to maintain a single repetitive exercise such as jogging in place or exercising to an aerobics video for an hour without getting bored—more power to them.

If you belong to a fitness facility, you may try the same principle as above by doing ten minutes on the stair machine, then ten minutes on the rowing machine, then ten minutes on the stationary bike. If you are seeking a full hour, try doubling the ten-minute periods to twenty minutes.

# CHAPTER 26

## WEIGHT TRAINING

The following weight training exercises are time efficient and cover all the major muscle groups of the body. There is no need to do lifts that isolate one muscle group such as abdominal crunches, bicep curls, or tricep extensions, etc., unless you like spending a lot of time in the gym. Doing lifts that isolate muscle groups are insignificant calorie burners. If you do have the time and want to work muscles individually, then more power to you. I prefer maximizing productivity in the least amount of time spent.

If you are just starting out, there is a "build up" phase meaning doing one set of eight to ten repetitions (reps) at each station. Reps are the process of repeating the same action over and over, in this case eight to ten times. A set is a group of the eight to ten reps. Two sets of eight to ten reps are executed in this way: Eight to ten reps, rest period, then eight to ten more reps.

## GETTING STARTED

Start out with a weight that feels very light to you. The second time you train the *same muscle group(s)*, (at least forty eight hours later), stay with one set of eight to ten reps but increase the weight a little. The third time you train the *same muscle group(s)*, do two sets of eight to ten reps with the amount of weight you trained the second time. The fourth time you train, do two sets of eight to ten reps with a little heavier weight. The fifth time, do three sets of eight to ten reps with the amount of weight that you trained with the fourth time. Keep progressing in this same fashion until you have built up to four sets of eight to ten reps per muscle group. Following this routine will enable you to exercise virtually pain free. If you happen to take a two-week or more break from **aerobic** or **anaerobic** exercise, it is probably a good idea to start over. Pain associated with exercise is one of the main reasons people drop their exercise programs. Below is a *prototype* for weight training you can follow, or you can be creative and make up your own:

## THE WORKOUT

| Day 1 | Day 2 | Day 3 | Day 4 | Day 5 | Day 6 | Day 7 |
|---|---|---|---|---|---|---|
| Total Body | Off | Total Body | Off | Total Body | Off | Total Body |

**And so on... OR...**

| Day 1 | Day 2 | Day 3 | Day 4 | Day 5 | Day 6 | Day 7 |
|---|---|---|---|---|---|---|
| Upper Body | Lower Body | Upper Body | Lower Body | Off | Off | Upper Body |

**And so on...**

134

In the future, as you get stronger, you will find that you can handle more weight for the four sets of eight to ten reps. When it starts getting too easy, increase the weight a little unless you are happy with your strength and/or how you look. You may also want to consider increasing the number of reps to the twelve to fifteen range if tone and definition are your major concerns. If you decide that tone and definition are your objectives, you may have to decrease the amount of weight you are using at each station. If strength and muscular size are your concern, aim for reps in the four to six range. You will need to increase the amount of weight you are using at each station if strength and muscular size are your objective. By working out with reps in the eight to ten range, you will be utilizing both the tone/definition and the strength/size systems.

## Good Form

All lifts should be executed with a *full range of motion* (total/complete flexion and total/complete extension). Throwing or swinging your body and/or weights to generate momentum should be avoided. You will see a lot of people in the gym throwing and swinging. You will also see those same people encouraging injuries as a result. Execute each lift by timing two seconds on all up phases and two seconds on all down phases (the two second rule). Each complete rep will take four seconds.

## Upper Body

The four exercises you are about to see develop all the major muscles of the upper body.

**The following pictures illustrate the Lat Pulldown exercise.**

135

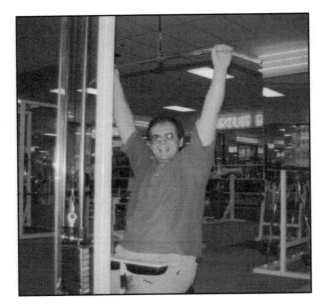

The start of the lift.

One-half rep
of the lift.

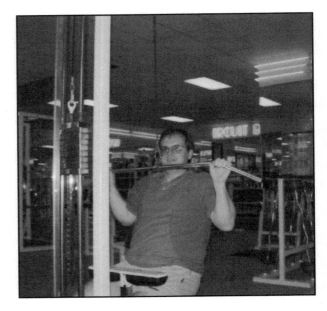

The top picture shows the start of the lift, and the picture below it shows one-half rep of the lift. It should take you two seconds from the start of the lift to the one-half rep position and another two seconds back to the start, constituting one full rep, a total of four seconds.

**The main muscle groups developed as a result of lat pulldown are:**
**Latissimus dorsi**—a large triangular muscle of which the apex is connected to the upper arm bones and fans out into a triangular shape connecting to the upper middle spine all the way down to the lower spine.
**Hand and wrist flexors**—anterior muscles of the lower arm that enable you to hold on to the bar.
**Rectus abdominus**—muscles of the front part of the abdomen sometimes called "abs," "six-pack," or "washboard."
**Biceps**—a two-headed muscle on the front of the upper arms.

**The following pictures illustrate the overhead press.**

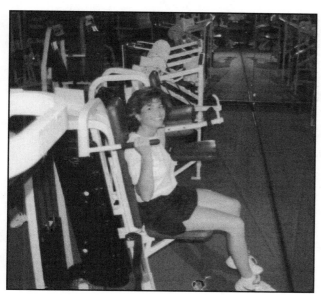

The start of the lift.

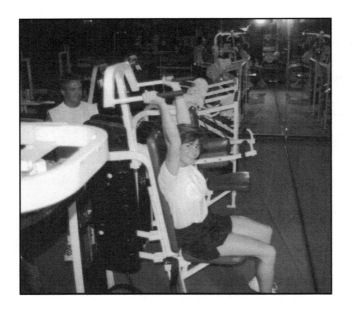

One-half rep
of the lift.

The picture on the previous page shows the start of the lift, and the above picture shows one half rep of the lift. The two-second rule also applies here.

**The main muscle groups developed as a result of overhead press are:**
**Anterior and medial deltoid**—two heads of the three-headed deltoid muscle covering the shoulder in a triangular fashion.
**Upper Trapezius**—a large flat muscle that forms a triangle from the back of the neck down to about the mid-back region. It then converges to the point of attachment at the back of the shoulder.
**Triceps**—a three-headed muscle on the back of the upper arm connecting it to the shoulder bones.

**The following pictures illustrate the row or bent-over row.**

The top picture shows the start of the lift, and the picture below

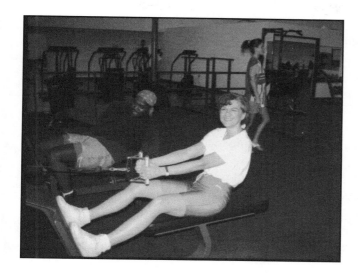

The start
of the lift.

One-half rep
of the lift.

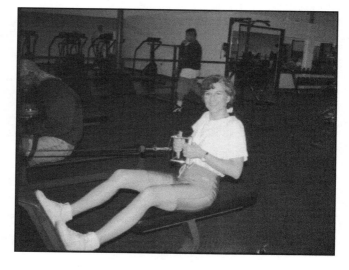

shows one-half rep of the lift.  The two-second rule also applies here.

**The main muscle groups developed as a result of the row or bent-over row are:**

**Teres major and minor**—muscles that lie beneath the trapezius connecting the shoulder blade to the upper part of the upper arm bone.
**Posterior deltoid**—the back part of the deltoid as explained in the overhead press previously.
**Rhomboid major and minor**—muscles of the back that lie under the middle part of the trapezius and pull the shoulder blades in toward the spine upon flexion.
**Middle/lower trapezius**—back and shoulder muscle explained in overhead press.
**Hand and wrist flexors**—explained previously in lat pulldown.
**Biceps**—explained previously in lat pulldown.
**Sacrospinalis**—muscles along the spine and lower back.
**Internal and external abdominal obliques**—muscles on the side of the abdomen.

**The following pictures illustrate the bench or chest press.**

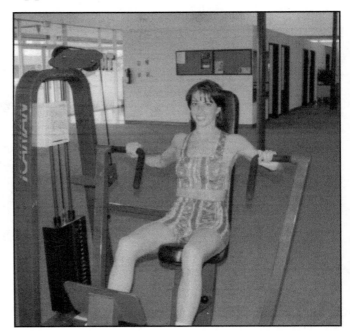

The start
of the lift.

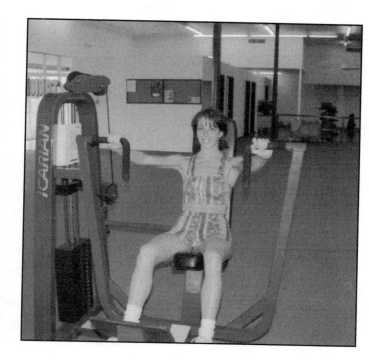

One-half rep
of the lift.

The picture on the previous page shows the start of the lift, and the picture above shows one-half rep of the lift. The two-second rule also applies here.

**The main muscle groups developed as a result of the bench or chest press are:**
**Pectoralis major and minor**—muscles of the chest connecting the middle part of the chest to the upper part of the upper arm bone.
**Anterior deltoid**—the front part of the deltoid muscle as explained in the overhead press.
**Triceps**—explained in overhead press previously.

## LOWER BODY

The two lifts you are about to see develop all the major muscle groups of the legs and buttocks.

**The following pictures illustrate the leg press.**

The picture below shows the start of the lift, and the picture on the following page shows one-half rep of the lift. The two-second rule also applies here.

**The main muscle groups developed as a result of the leg press are:**
**Gluteus maximus, gluteus medius, and gluteus minimus**—muscles of the buttocks and outer hip.
**Semimembranosis, semitendinosus, and biceps femorus (hamstrings)**—muscles of the back of the thigh.

The start
of the lift.

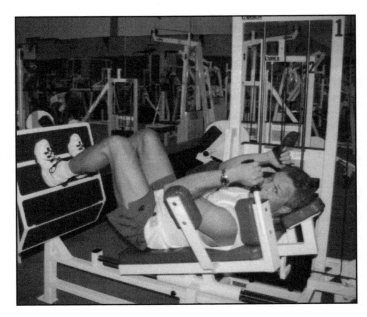

142

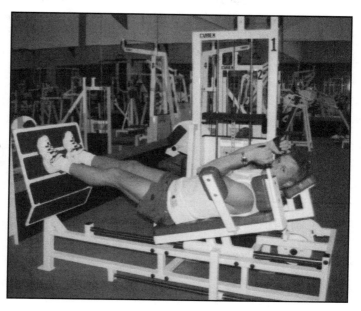

One-half rep
of the lift.

**Rectus femorus, vastus intermedius, vastus medialis, and vastus lateralis (quadraceps)**—the four main muscles of the front of the thigh.
**Sartorius**—the longest muscle in the body. It wraps around the front of the thigh.
**Gracilis, adductor magnus, adductor brevis, and adductor longus (adductors)**—muscles of the inner thigh.

Vary your foot placement. As you build up to four sets, do one set with your feet together in the middle and one set with your feet together in the high middle position. The other two sets should be done with your feet in the wide middle and wide high positions.

**The following pictures illustrate calf raises.**

143

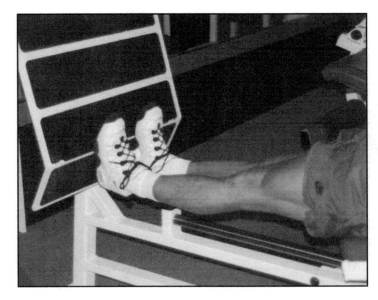

The start
of the lift.

One-half rep
of the lift.

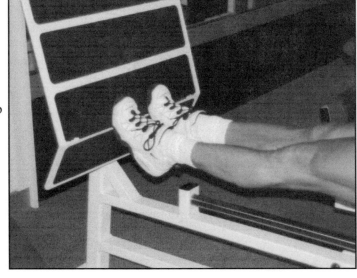

The top picture shows the start of the lift, and the picture below it shows one-half rep of the lift. The two-second rule also applies here.

**The main muscle groups developed as a result of calf raises are:**
**Gastrocnemius (calf)**—the main muscle in the back of the lower leg.
**Soleus**—the muscle that lies under the gastrocnemius.

## SEEK VARIETY AND EMANCIPATE

There are many variations to all the lifts you have read about. For example, as you progress, you may want to vary your grip on the lat pulldown or do two sets of overhead press with dumbbells and two sets on the machine as pictured previously, etc.

You do not need to become a slave to the gym. Doing abdomen crunches until you are "blue in the face" burns an insignificant number of calories and will not reveal your "abs" if you have a significant layer of fat covering them up. Shed the fat via calorie deficits, and you will discover "abs" without performing exclusive abdomen exercises. The lat pulldown (page 136) and the rowing machine (page 149) do a great job on the "abs."

The same principle applies to individual bicep and tricep exercises (bicep curls and tricep extensions burn an insignificant number of calories while adding time to your workout). By doing four sets of lat pulldown and four sets of bent row, your biceps are working eight sets. Triceps are involved with other muscle groups while performing overhead and bench press.

Give yourself fifty to ninety seconds in between each set to allow your muscles to recover. There are other techniques called "super sets, pyrimiding," etc., that do not allow rest periods. They are reserved for the seasoned veteran or you after about six consistent months of following this plan. Ask a competent/qualified personal trainer about other training methods if you decide to try something new.

# PERSONAL TRAINERS?

Hiring a personal trainer or checking out other books on lifting may be a good idea to show you variations, make sure your form is good, or just to show you new lifts. Beware though, there are many unqualified trainers who can do more harm than good. Anyone who looks "buff" and has taken a weekend crash course is not necessarily qualified. Look for someone who is personable with at least a bachelor's degree in some type of exercise science.

**Beware of trainers who:**
1. Use the "no-pain, no-gain" philosophy.
2. Suggest swinging the weights or your body in any manner.
3. Ask you to do any abdominal exercise that compromises your lower back such as sit-ups with straight legs or the exercise called "straight leg lifts." Crunches are fine if the thigh is perpendicular to the floor while lying on your back and you do not mind being a slave to the gym.
4. Ask you to pick up anything via bending over rather than kneeling down.
5. Leave you unattended or frequently divert their attention away from you during your training session.
6. Use negative reinforcement.

# CHAPTER 27

## CALORIES....BURN 'EM THE OLD FASHIONED WAY!

The chart on the following page (Table 27-1) lists various forms of exercise that burn varying amounts of calories *per hour.* Your personal BMR number from page 42 already accounts for basic everyday sedentary activities like sleeping, brushing your teeth, driving, sitting, walking around, and other *non-exercising* activities. As you browse through the numbers, you will notice there are some activities very close to others. Equipment such as Stairmaster, Schwinn Airdyne, Life Cycles, and others have the capability of telling you how many calories you burn, so I did not list them.

There are many other activities I have not listed: badminton (recreation), baseball, softball, dancing, hiking with a backpack, horseback riding, canoeing (3.5 mph), rollerblading (moderate), ice and roller skating (moderate), snow and water-skiing (moderate), and volleyball (moderate). You can use the *low impact aerobic dance numbers* for the activities listed above. For archery, bowling, boxing, calisthenics, fencing (moderate), football (moderate), canoeing (3 mph), horseback riding (walk), horseshoe pitching, and sailing, use the *cycling (6 mph) numbers.* For badminton (competition), fencing (vigorous), handball, mountain climbing, rollerblading (vigorous), ice and roller skating (vigorous), snow skiing (vigorous), squash, and volleyball (vigorous), use the *aerobic dance (high impact) numbers.* For football (vigorous) and water-skiing (vigorous), use the *weight training numbers.*

These numbers have been formulated to account for brief rest periods such as the fifty to ninety seconds between sets while weight training. If you spend a lot of time talking to friends in between sets (longer than fifty to ninety seconds), you should consider the extra time in your calculations. The same goes for excessive rest periods in all the activities listed. For example: a couple of five-minute breaks during basketball or tennis is insignificant. A couple of ten-minute breaks could affect the numbers significantly. As you keep playing with the numbers regularly, you will depend less and less on the following table (Table 27-1).

## Table 27-1

| Body Weight (lbs.) | 90 | 100 | 110 | 120 | 130 | 140 | 150 | 160 | 170 | 180 |
|---|---|---|---|---|---|---|---|---|---|---|
| | | | | | Calories burned per hour | | | | | |
| **Aerobic Dance or Step Aerobics** | | | | | | | | | | |
| Low Impact | 204 | 228 | 246 | 274 | 300 | 324 | 336 | 366 | 384 | 408 |
| High Impact | 354 | 384 | 420 | 456 | 512 | 558 | 594 | 624 | 660 | 696 |
| **Basketball** | | | | | | | | | | |
| Moderate | 252 | 276 | 300 | 335 | 373 | 402 | 426 | 450 | 474 | 498 |
| Competition | 354 | 390 | 426 | 468 | 518 | 564 | 600 | 636 | 667 | 702 |
| **Cycling** | | | | | | | | | | |
| Level 6 m.p.h. | 180 | 198 | 216 | 234 | 270 | 288 | 306 | 324 | 336 | 354 |
| Level 13 m.p.h. | 384 | 426 | 462 | 508 | 566 | 612 | 648 | 684 | 726 | 762 |
| **Golf** | | | | | | | | | | |
| Walk w/bag | 198 | 216 | 234 | 255 | 283 | 312 | 330 | 348 | 366 | 384 |
| Riding/playing from cart ............insignificant | | | | | | | | | | |
| **Martial Arts** | 462 | 510 | 552 | 610 | 680 | 732 | 780 | 822 | 870 | 912 |
| **Racquetball** | | | | | | | | | | |
| Leisure | 312 | 360 | 402 | 460 | 530 | 582 | 630 | 672 | 720 | 762 |
| Competitive | 462 | 510 | 552 | 610 | 680 | 732 | 780 | 822 | 870 | 912 |
| **Rowing Machine** | | | | | | | | | | |
| Slow | 180 | 198 | 216 | 244 | 270 | 288 | 306 | 324 | 336 | 360 |
| Fast | 492 | 540 | 588 | 646 | 722 | 780 | 828 | 876 | 924 | 972 |
| **Running** | | | | | | | | | | |
| Averaging: | | | | | | | | | | |
| 11 min. /mile | 384 | 426 | 462 | 508 | 566 | 612 | 648 | 684 | 726 | 762 |
| 8.5 min./mile | 492 | 540 | 588 | 646 | 722 | 780 | 828 | 876 | 924 | 972 |
| 7 min./mile | 558 | 612 | 667 | 774 | 834 | 888 | 942 | 996 | 1050 | 1134 |
| 5 min./mile | 708 | 780 | 846 | 928 | 1046 | 1122 | 1194 | 1260 | 1332 | 1398 |
| **Soccer** | 324 | 354 | 384 | 414 | 470 | 510 | 540 | 576 | 606 | 636 |
| **Swimming** | | | | | | | | | | |
| Slow Crawl | 204 | 228 | 246 | 274 | 300 | 324 | 336 | 366 | 384 | 408 |
| Fast Crawl | 384 | 426 | 462 | 508 | 566 | 612 | 648 | 684 | 726 | 762 |
| **Tennis** | | | | | | | | | | |
| Recreation | 252 | 276 | 300 | 335 | 373 | 402 | 426 | 450 | 474 | 498 |
| Competition | 354 | 390 | 426 | 468 | 518 | 564 | 600 | 636 | 667 | 702 |
| **Walking** | | | | | | | | | | |
| Avg. pace 3 m.p.h. | 180 | 198 | 216 | 234 | 270 | 288 | 306 | 324 | 336 | 354 |
| Brisk pace 4 m.p.h. | 204 | 228 | 246 | 274 | 300 | 324 | 336 | 366 | 384 | 408 |
| **Weight Training** | 288 | 312 | 330 | 348 | 426 | 462 | 480 | 498 | 540 | 558 |

Table 27-1 (continued)

| Body Weight (lbs.) | 190 | 200 | 210 | 220 | 230 | 240 | 250 | 260 | 270 | 280 | 290 | 300 |
|---|---|---|---|---|---|---|---|---|---|---|---|---|
| | | | | | | Calories burned per hour | | | | | | |
| **Aerobic Dance or Step Aerobics** | | | | | | | | | | | | |
| Low Impact | 426 | 454 | 476 | 498 | 528 | 546 | 564 | 588 | 606 | 624 | 645 | 667 |
| High Impact | 726 | 772 | 824 | 864 | 900 | 936 | 966 | 1002 | 1038 | 1074 | 1110 | 1132 |
| **Basketball** | | | | | | | | | | | | |
| Moderate | 528 | 552 | 590 | 624 | 648 | 672 | 696 | 726 | 750 | 774 | 799 | 825 |
| Competition | 738 | 784 | 830 | 876 | 900 | 912 | 978 | 1014 | 1050 | 1086 | 1122 | 1159 |
| **Cycling** | | | | | | | | | | | | |
| Level 6 m.p.h. | 372 | 390 | 426 | 444 | 462 | 480 | 498 | 516 | 534 | 552 | 573 | 594 |
| Level 13 m.p.h. | 804 | 850 | 902 | 954 | 990 | 1026 | 1068 | 1104 | 1140 | 1176 | 1212 | 1250 |
| **Golf** | | | | | | | | | | | | |
| Walk w/bag | 402 | 436 | 452 | 480 | 498 | 516 | 540 | 558 | 576 | 600 | 624 | 650 |
| Riding/playing from cart..............insignificant | | | | | | | | | | | | |
| **Martial Arts** | 960 | 1012 | 1082 | 1140 | 1182 | 1230 | 1272 | 1320 | 1362 | 1410 | 1458 | 1506 |
| **Racquetball** | | | | | | | | | | | | |
| Leisure | 810 | 862 | 932 | 990 | 1032 | 1080 | 1122 | 1170 | 1212 | 1260 | 1308 | 1356 |
| Competitive | 960 | 1012 | 1082 | 1140 | 1182 | 1230 | 1272 | 1320 | 1362 | 1410 | 1458 | 1506 |
| **Rowing Machine** | | | | | | | | | | | | |
| Slow | 372 | 390 | 426 | 444 | 462 | 480 | 498 | 516 | 534 | 552 | 573 | 594 |
| Fast | 1020 | 1078 | 1154 | 1212 | 1260 | 1308 | 1356 | 1404 | 1452 | 1500 | 1548 | 1596 |
| **Running** | | | | | | | | | | | | |
| Averaging: | | | | | | | | | | | | |
| 11 min. /mile | 804 | 850 | 902 | 954 | 990 | 1026 | 1068 | 1104 | 1140 | 1176 | 1212 | 1250 |
| 8.5 min./mile | 1020 | 1078 | 1154 | 1212 | 1260 | 1308 | 1356 | 1404 | 1452 | 1500 | 1548 | 1596 |
| 7 min./mile | 1158 | 1222 | 1316 | 1380 | 1434 | 1488 | 1542 | 1596 | 1650 | 1704 | 1758 | 1812 |
| 5 min./mile | 1470 | 1546 | 1664 | 1746 | 1812 | 1884 | 1950 | 2022 | 2094 | 2160 | 2226 | 2290 |
| **Soccer** | 667 | 706 | 738 | 784 | 830 | 876 | 900 | 912 | 978 | 1014 | 1050 | 1086 |
| **Swimming** | | | | | | | | | | | | |
| Slow Crawl | 426 | 454 | 476 | 498 | 528 | 546 | 564 | 588 | 606 | 624 | 645 | 667 |
| Fast Crawl | 804 | 850 | 902 | 954 | 990 | 1026 | 1068 | 1104 | 1140 | 1176 | 1212 | 1250 |
| **Tennis** | | | | | | | | | | | | |
| Recreation | 528 | 552 | 590 | 624 | 648 | 672 | 696 | 726 | 750 | 774 | 799 | 825 |
| Competition | 738 | 784 | 830 | 876 | 900 | 912 | 978 | 1014 | 1050 | 1086 | 1122 | 1159 |
| **Walking** | | | | | | | | | | | | |
| Avg. pace, 3 mph | 372 | 390 | 426 | 444 | 462 | 480 | 498 | 516 | 534 | 552 | 573 | 594 |
| Brisk pace, 4 mph | 426 | 454 | 476 | 498 | 528 | 546 | 564 | 588 | 606 | 624 | 645 | 667 |
| **Weight Training** | 600 | 642 | 667 | 702 | 732 | 762 | 793 | 810 | 834 | 864 | 894 | 924 |

# BIBLIOGRAPHY

## SECTION I

**Burke, L.M. et al.** "Muscle glycogen storage after prolonged exercise: effect of glycemic index of carbohydrate feedings." *Journal of Applied Physiology*, 1993, 75(2): 1019.

**Coyle, E.F. and Coyle, E.** "Carbohydrates that speed recovery from training." *Physiology of Sports Medicine*, 1993, 21:111.

**Price, T.B. et al.** "Human muscle glycogen resynthesis after exercise: Insulin dependent and independent phases." *Journal of Applied Physiology*, 1994, 76(1):104.

**Frayn, K.N. et al.** "Effect of diet on human adipose tissue metabolism." *Proceedings of the Nutrition Society*, 1992, 51:409.

**Jefferson, L.S.** "Role of insulin in the regulation of protein synthesis." *Diabetes, 1980*, 29:487.

**Jequier, E.** "Carbohydrates as a source of energy." *American Journal of Clinical Nutrition*, 1994, 59:682S.

**Johnson, T.R. and Ilan, J.** "Expression of IGF-1 in liver." Molecular and Cellular Biology of Insulin-Like Growth Factors and Their Receptors, 1989, 129.

**Scott, C.D. and Baxter, R.C.** "Production of insulin-like growth factor 1 and its binding protein in rat hepatocyte cultures from diabetic and insulin-treated diabetic rats." *Endocrinology*, 1986, 119:2346.

151

**Taylor, R., Price T.B., Katz, L.D. et al.** "Direct measurement of change in muscle glycogen concentration after a mixed meal in normal subjects." *American Journal of Physiology*, 265 (1993): E224.

**Colgan, M.** *Optimum Sports Nutrition.* Advanced Research Press, 1993.

**Daughaday, W.H.** *Endocrine Control of Growth.* New York: Elsevier, 1981.

Weigle, DS. *Diabetes*, 1987; 36:764.

**Salmon, W.D. and Daughaday, W.H.** "A hormonally controlled serum factor which stimulates sulfate incorporation by cartilage in vitro." *Journal of Laboratory Clinical Investigation*, 1957; 49:825.

**Laron, A. et al.** *Evaluation of Growth Hormone Secretion.* Basel Karger Publishing, 1983.

**Rolls, B.J.** "Carbohydrates, fats and satiety." *American Journal of Clinical Nutrition* 61 (supple.): 960s, 1995.

**Pizza, F.X., Flynn, M.G., and Duscha, B.D. et al.** "A carbohydrate loading regimen improves high intensity, short duration exercise performance." *International Journal of Sport Nutrition*, 1995, 5: 110.

**Lee, I.M. and Paffenbarger, R.S., Jr**. "Change in body weight and longevity." *Journal of American Medical Association*, Oct 21, 1992:268 (15): 2045.

**Higgins, M., Kannel, W., Garrison R., Pinsky J., and Stokes, J.** "Hazards of obesity - the Framingham experience." *Acta Medical Scandinavica, Supplement*, 1988, 723:23.

**Higgins, M., D'Agostino, R., Kannel, W., and Cobb, J.** "Benefits and adverse effects of weight loss. The Framingham Study." *Annals of Internal Medicine* (US), Oct 1, 1993, 119 (7Pt2):758.

**Willett, W.C., Manson, J.E., Stampfer, M.J., Colditz, G.A., Rosner, B., and Speizer, F.E.** "Weight, weight change, and coronary heart disease in women. Risk within the normal weight range." *Journal of American Medical Association*, (US), Feb. 8, 1995, 273 (6):461.

**Kuller, L.H.** "Eating fat or being fat and risk of cardiovascular disease and cancer in women." *Annals of Epidemiology*, (US), March 1994, 4 (2):119.

**Hammer, R.L; Barrier, C.A; Roundy, E.S et al.** "Calorie-restricted low-fat diet and exercise in obese women." *American Journal of Clinical*

*Nutrition*, 1989, 49:77.

**Kim, M.J., Roecker, E.B., and Weindruch, R.** "Influences of aging and dietary restriction on red blood cell density profiles and antioxidant enzyme activities in rhesus monkeys." *Experimental Gerontology*, (England), Nov.-Dec., 1993, 28(6):515.

**Lane, M.A., Ingram, D.K., Cutler, R.G., Knapka, J.J., Barnard, D.E., and Roth, G.S.** "Dietary restriction in nonhuman primates: progress report on the NIA study." *Annals of New York Academy of Science* (US), Dec. 26, 1992, 673:36.

**Kemnitz, J.W., Weindruch, R., Roecker, E.B., Crawford, K., Kaufman, P.L., and Ershler, W.B.** "Dietary restriction of adult male rhesus monkeys: Design, methodology and preliminary findings from the first year of study." *Journal of Gerontology*, (US), Jan., 1993, 48 (1):17.

**Rolls, B.J.** "Carbohydrates, fats, and satiety." *American Journal of Clinical Nutrition*, 1995, 61 (suppl.):960s.

**Froesch, et al.** "Metabolic and therapeutic effects of insulin-like growth factor-1." *Hormone Research*, 1994, 2:66.

**Ling, et al.** "IGF-1 alters energy expenditure and protein metabolism during parenteral feeding in rats." *American Journal of Clinical Nutrition*, 1995, 61:116.

**Zapf,** "Insulin-like growth factors/somatomedins: Structure, secretion, biological actions and physiological roles." *Hormone Research*, 1986, 24:121.

**Millward, D.J., Rivers, H.P.W.** "The need for indispensable amino acids: The concept of the anabolic drive." *Diabetes Melab Review*, 1989, 5:191.

**Laron, A. et al.** *Evaluation of Growth Hormone Secretion.* Basel Karger Publishing, 1983.

**Miller, C.J., Baggett, J.R., Morris, M., Stewart, P., Lewis, W., Strickland, M., and Bishop, M. et al.** *Laboratory Manual for Health Concepts of Physical Activity.* Kendall/Hunt Publishing Co., 1986, 6:33.

**Bailey, C.** *The New Fit or Fat.* Houghton Mifflin Co., 1991, p.143.

**Siri, W.** "The Gross Composition of the Body." In: Lawrence, J. and Tobias, C. (editors), *Advances in Biological and Medical Physics.* 1956, Academic Press, New York.

**Jackson, A. and Pollack, M.** "Practical Assessment of Body Composition." *The Physician and Sports Medicine.* May, 1985, 13:86.


## SECTION II
**Cort,** "Antioxidant activity of tocopherols, ascorbyl palmitate, and ascorbic acid and their mode of action." *Journal of the American Oil Chemists Society.* 1974, 51:321.

**Hendler, S.** *The Doctors Vitamin and Mineral Encyclopedia.* 1990, p.432 and 395. Simon and Schuster, New York.

**Pearson, D. and Shaw, S.** *Life Extension.* 1983, pgs. 306, 390, 485 and 618. Warner Books, New York.

**Colgan, M.** *Optimum Sports Nutrition.* 1993, p.217. Advanced Research Press, New York.

**National Research Council,** *Recommended Dietary Allowances.* 1989, 10th edition, 176. National Academy Press, Washington, DC.

**Kronhausen, E. and Kronhausen, P.** *Formula For Life.* 1989, p.44. William Morrow, New York.


### The carotenoid complex
**Kummet, T., et al.** "Vitamin A. Evidence for its preventive role in human cancer." *Nutrition and Cancer.* 1983, 5:96.

**Menkes, M.S., and Comstock, G.W.** "Vitamin A and E and lung cancer." *American Journal of Epidemiology.* 1984, 120:491.

**Menkes, M.S., Comstock, G.W. et al.** "Serum beta carotene, vitamins A and E, selenium, and the risk of lung cancer." *New England Journal of Medicine.* 1986, 315(20):1250.

**Cutler, Richard G.** "Carotenoids and retinol: their possible importance in determining longevity of primate species." *Proceedings of the National Academy of Science.* USA, 1984, 81:7629.

**Maugh, T.H.** "Vitamin A: potential protection from carcinogens." *Science.* 1974, 186:1198.

**Alexander, M., Neumark, H., and Miller, R.G.** "Oral beta carotene can increase the number of OKT4+ cells in human blood." *Immunology*

*Letters.* 1985, 9:221.

**Bjelke, E.** "Dietary vitamin A and human lung cancer." *International Journal of Cancer.* 1975, 15:561.

**Bendich, A.** "The safety of beta carotene." *Nutrition and Cancer.* 1988, 11:207.

**Bendich, A.** "Carotenoids and the immune response." *Journal of Nutrition.* 1989, 119:112.

**Bendich, A. and Langseth, L.** "Safety of vitamin A." *American Journal of Clinical Nutrition.* 1989, 49:358.

**Modan, B., Chuckle, H., and Lubin, F.** "Retinol, carotene, and cancer." *International Journal of Cancer.* 1981, 28:421.

**Gerber, L.E. and Erdman, J.W. Jr.** "Effect of dietary retinyl acetate, beta carotene, and retinoic acid on wound healing in rats." *Journal of Nutrition.* 1982, 112:1555.

**Shekelle, R.B., Liu, S., Raynor, W.J., et al.** "Dietary vitamin A and risk of cancer in Western Electric study." *Lancet.* 1981, 2:1185.

**Goldfarb, M.T., et al.** "Topical tretinoin therapy: its use in photoaged skin." *Journal of the American Academy of Dermatology.* 1989, 645.

**Sporn, M.B., Dunlop, N.M., Dewton, D.L., et al.** "Prevention of chemical carcinogenesis by vitamin A and its synthetic analogs (retinoids)." *Federation Proceedings.* 1980, 35:1332.

**Krinsky, N.I.** "Carotenoids and cancer in animal models." *Journal of Nutrition.* 1989, 119:123.

**Peto, R., Doll, R., Buckley, J.D., et al.** "Can dietary beta carotene materially reduce human cancer rates?" *Nature.* 1981, 290:201.

**Kune, G.A., et al.** "Serum levels of beta carotene, vitamin A, and zinc in male lung cancer cases and controls." *Nutrition and Cancer.* 1989, 12:169.

**Hicks, R.M.** "The scientific basis for regarding vitamin A and its analogs as anti-carcinogenic agents." *Proceedings of the Nutrition Society.* 1983, 42:83.

**Levenson, S.M., et al.** "Supplemental vitamin A prevents the acute radiation-induced defect in wound healing." *Annals of Surgery.* 1984, 200:494.

**Lowe, N.J., Lazarus, V., and Matt, L.** "Systemic retinoid therapy for psoriasis." *Journal of the American Academy of Dermatology.* 1988, 19:186.

**Ziegler, R.G.** "A review of epidemiologic evidence that carotenoids reduce the risk of cancer." *Journal of Nutrition.* 1989, 119:116.

**Mickshe, M., et al.** "Stimulation of immune system response in lung cancer patients by vitamin A therapy." *Oncology.* 1977, 34:234-238.

**Weiss, J.S. et al.** "Topical tretinoin improves photoaged skin: A double blind, vehicle controlled study." *Journal of the American Medical Association.* 1988, 259:527.

**Salonen, J.T. et al.** "Risk of cancer in relation to serum concentrations of selenium and vitamins A and E: Matched case-control analysis of prospective data." *British Medical Journal.* 1985, 290:417.

### Grape seed extract

**Rao, C. Rao, V., and Steinman, B.** "Influence of bioflavonoids on the metabolism and crosslinking of collagen." *Italian Journal of Biochemistry.* 1981, 30, p.259.

**Cody, V. et al.** *Plant Bioflavonoids in Biology and Medicine.* 1986, 1988. Volumes 1 and 2. New York, New York, Alan Liss.

**Colgin. M.** *The New Nutrition.* 1994, p.136. C. I. Publications, Encinitas, Ca.

**Gissen, A.** "Grape seed extract, Pycnogenols, Pycnogenol and Proanthocyanidins." *Nutritional News.* March, 1995, 9:2.

### Bilberry extract

**Bever, B., and Zahnd, G.** "Plants with oral hypoglycemic action," *Quarterly Journal of Crude Drug Research.* 1979, 17, p. 139.

**Allen, F.** "Blueberry leaf extract: physiologic and clinical properties in relation to carbohydrate metabolism," *Journal of The American Medical Association.* 1927, 89, p.1577.

**Gabor, M.** "Pharmacologic effects of flavonoids on blood vessels," *Angiologica.* 1972, 9, p.355.

**Kahnau, J.** "The flavonoids. A class of semi-essential food components: their role in human nutrition," *World Review Nutrition and Dietetics.* 1976, 24, p. 117.

**Havsteen, B.** "Flavonoids, a class of natural products of high pharmacological potency," *Biochemical Pharmacology*. 1983, 32, p. 1141.

**Middleton, E.** "The flavonoids," *Trends in Pharmaceutical Science*. 1984, 5, p. 335.

### Milk thistle extract (silymarin)

**Hikino, H., Kiso, Y., Wagner, H., and Fiebig, M.** "Antihepatotoxic of flavonolignans from silybum marianum fruits," *Planta Medica*, 1984, 50, p. 248.

**Agarwal, R., Katiyar, S., Lundgren, D., and Mukhtar, H.** "Inhibitory effect of silymarin, an antihepatotoxic flavonoid, on 12-0-tetradecanoylphorbol-13-acetate-induced epidermal ornithine decarboxylase activity and mRNA in sencar mice," *Carcinogenesis* (United Kingdom). 1994, 15, p.1099.

**Salmi, H., and Sarna, S.** "Effect of silymarin on chemical, functional, and morphological alteration of the liver. A double-blind placebo controlled study," *Scandinavian Journal of Gastroenterology*. 1982, 17, p.417.

**Canni, F., Bartolucci, A., Cristallini, E., et al.** "Use of silymarin in the treatment of alcoholic hepatic stenosis," *Clinical Therapeutics*. 1985, 114, p. 307.

**Wagner, H.** "Plant constituents with antihepatotoxic activity," in Beal J. and Richard, E., (eds.) *Natural Products as Medicinal Agents*, Hippokrates-Verlag, Stuttgart, 1981.

### Vitamin Bl (thiamin)

**Kent, S.** *Your Personal Life Extension Program*. 1985, p.141. William Morrow and Co., Inc. New York.

**Kronhausen, E., and Kronhausen, P.** *Formula for Life*. 1989, p.135. William Morrow and Co., Inc. New York.

**Katz, D., et al.** "Intestinal absorption of thiamin from yeast-containing sorghum beer." *American Journal of Clinical Nutrition*. 1985, 42:666.

**Pearson, D., and Shaw, S.** *Life Extension*. 1982, pgs. 88, 280-281, 264, and 373. Warner Books, Inc. New York.

**Mandel, H. et al.** "Thiamin-dependent beriberi in the thiamin responsive anemia syndrome." *New England Journal of Medicine*. 1984, 311:836.

**Skelton, W.P. and Skelton, N.K.** "Thiamin deficiency neuropathy: It's still common today." *Postgraduate Medicine.* 1989, 85(8):301.
**Rosenbaum, M.E. and Bosco, D.** *Super Supplements.* 1987, pgs. 96 and 214. Signet Books, New York.

### Vitamin B2 (riboflavin)
**Belko, A.Z., et al.** "Effects of exercise on riboflavin requirements of young women." *American Journal of Clinical Nutrition.* 1983, 37:509.
**Belko, A.Z., et al.** "Effects of aerobic exercise and weight loss on riboflavin requirements of moderately obese, marginally deficient young women." *American Journal of Clinical Nutrition.* 1984, 40:553.
**Munoz, N. et al.** "Effect of riboflavin, retinol, and zinc on micronuclei of buccal mucosa and of esophagus: A randomized double-blind intervention study in China." *Journal of the National Cancer Institute.* 1987, 79:687.
**Powers, H.J., Wright, A.J.A., and Fairweather-Tait, J.J.** "The effect of riboflavin deficiency in rats on the absorption and distribution of iron." *British Journal of Nutrition.* 1988, 59:381.

### Vitamin B3 (niacin, nicotinic acid, or niacinimide)
**Canner, P.L., et al.** "Fifteen year mortality in coronary drug project patients: Long term benefit with niacin." *Journal of the American College of Cardiology.* 1986, 8:1245.
**Hawkins, D., Pauling, L.** *Orthomolecular Psychiatry.* 1973, pgs. 667. W.H. Freeman and Co., San Francisco.
**Miettinen, T.A., et al.** "Glucose tolerance and plasma insulin in man during acute and chronic administration of nicotinic acid." *Acta Medica Scandinavica.* 1969, 186:247.
**Carlson, L.A., Hamsten, A., and Asplund, A.** "Pronounced lowering of serum levels of lipoprotein Lp(a) in hyperlipidemic subjects treated with nicotinic acid." *Journal of Internal Medicine.* 1989, 226:271.
**Hoffer, A.** "Treatment of arthritis by nicotinic acid and nicotinamide." *Canadian Medical Association Journal.* 1959, 81:235.
**Hoffer, A.** *Niacin Therapy in Psychiatry.* 1962, Charles C. Thomas, Springfield, Ill.

**Hoffer, A., Walker, M.** *Orthomolecular Nutrition: New Lifestyle for Super Good Health.* 1978, Keats Publishing, New Canaan, Conn.
**The Coronary Drug Project Research Group,** "Clofibrate and niacin in coronary heart disease." *Journal of the American Medical Association.* 1975, 231(4):360.
**Knopp, R.H. et al.** "Contrasting effects of unmodified and time release forms of niacin on lipoproteins in hyperlipidemic subjects: Clue to mechanism of action of niacin." *Metabolism.* 1985, 34:442.
**Yovos, J.G., et al.** "Effects of nicotinic acid therapy on plasma lipoproteins and very low density lipoprotein apoprotein C subspecies in hyperlipoproteinerria." *Journal of Clinical Endocrinology and Metabolism.* 1982, 54:1210.
**Luria, M.H.** "Effect of low-dose niacin on high density lipoprotein cholesterol and total cholesterol/high density lipoprotein cholesterol ratio." *Archives of Internal Medicine.* 1988, 148:2493.
**Grundy, Scott M., et al.** "Influence of nicotinic acid on metabolism of cholesterol and triglycerides in man." *Journal of Lipid Research.* 1981, 22:24.
**Kaufman, W.** "Niacinimide therapy for joint mobility: Therapeutic reversal of a common clinical manifestation of the "normal" aging process." *Connecticut State Medical Journal.* 1953, 17:584.
**Kaufman, W.** "The use of vitamin therapy to reverse certain concomitants of aging." *Journal of the American Geriatrics Society.* 1955, 3:927.
**Kaufman, W.** "Niacinimide, a most neglected vitamin." *International Academy of Preventive Medicine.* 1983, 8:5.

### Vitamin B5 (pantothenic acid or calcium pantothenate)
**Ralli, E.P. and Dumm, M.E.** "Relation of pantothentic acid to adrenal cortical function." *Vitamins and Hormones.* 1953, 11:133.
**Barton-Wright, E.C. and Elliot, W.A.** "The pantothentic acid metabolism of rheumatoid arthritis." Lancet. 1963, 862.
**General Practitioner Research Group,** "Calcium pantothenate in arthritic conditions." *Practitioner.* 1980, 224:208.
**Litoff, D. Scherzer, H. and Harrison, J.** "Effects of pantothentic acid supplementation on human exercise." *Medicine and Science in Sports*

*and Exercise.* 1985, 17:287.

**Kronhausen, E., and Kronhausen, P.** *Formula for Life.* 1989, pgs.137-140. William Morrow and Co., Inc. New York.

**Nice, C. et al.** "The effects of pantothentic acid on human exercise capacity." *Journal of Sports Medicine.* 1984, 24:26.

**Goodman, L.S., and Gilman, A.G.** *The Pharmacological Basis of Therapeutics.* 1985, p.1572. Macmillan, New York.

**Pauling, L.** *How To Live Longer and Feel Better.* 1986, p.88. W.H. Freeman and Co. New York.

### Vitamin B6 (pyridoxine)

**Ellis, J.M.** *The Doctor Who Looked at Hands.* 1966. Vantage Press, New York.

**Ellis, J.M., Presley, J.** *Vitamin B6, The Doctor's Report.* 1973. Harper and Row, New York.

**Ellis, J.M. et al.** "Response of Vitamin B6 deficiency and the carpal tunnel syndrome to pyridoxine." *Proceedings of the National Academy of Science.* 1982, 79:7494.

**Ellis, J.M.** *Free of Pain: A Proven and Inexpensive Treatment for Specific Types of Rheumatism.* 1983. Southwest Publishing, Brownsville and Dallas, Texas.

**Ellis, J.M.** "Treatment of carpal tunnel syndrome with vitamin B6." *Southern Medical Journal.* 1987, 80:882.

**Abraham, G.E., and Hargrove J.** "Effect of vitamin B6 on premenstrual symptomatology in women with premenstrual tension syndromes: A double-blind crossover study." *Infertility.* 1980, 3:155.

**Kasden, M.L., and James, C.J.** "Carpal tunnel syndrome and vitamin B6." *Plastic and Reconstructive Surgery.* 1987, 80:882.

**Rinehart, J.F., and Greenberg, L.D.** "Arteriosclerotic lesions in pyridoxine deficient monkeys." *American Journal of Pathology.* 1969, 25:481.

**DiSorbo, D.M., and Nathanson, L.** "High dose pyridoxal supplemented culture medium inhibits the growth of a human malignant melanoma cell line." *Nutrition and Cancer.* 1983, 5(1):10.

**DiSorbo, D.M., Wagner, R. Jr., and Nathanson, L.** "In vivo and in vitro inhibition of B16 melanoma growth by B6." *Nutrition and Cancer.* 1985, 7:43.

**Baumblat, M.J., and Winston F.** "Pyridoxine and the pill." *Lancet.* 1970, 1:832.

**Adams, P.W. et al.** "Influence of oral contraceptives, pyridoxine, and tryptophan on carbohydrate metabolism." *Lancet.* 1976, 1:759.

**Schaumberg, H. et al.** "Sensory neuropathy from pyridoxine abuse." *New England Journal of Medicine.* 1983, 309:445.

### Vitamin B12 (cobalamin)

**Goodwin, J.S., et al.** "Association between nutritional status and cognitive functioning in a healthy elderly population." *Journal of the American Medical Association.* 1983, 249:2917.

**Anonymous,** "Vitamin B12 confirmed as effective sulfite allergy blocker." *Allergy Observer.* March-April 1987, 4(2):1.

**Campbell, M. et al.** "Rastafarianism and the vegans syndrome." *British Medical Journal.* 1982, 285:1617.

**Lindenbaum, J., et al.** "Neuropsychiatric disorders caused by cobalamin deficiency in the absence of anemia or macrocytosis." *New England Journal of Medicine.* 1988, 318:1720.

**Beck, W.S.** "Cobalamin and the nervous system (editorial)." *New England Journal of Medicine.* 1988, 318:1752.

**Jacobsen, D.W., Simon, R.A., and Singh, M.** "Sulfite oxidase deficiency and cobalamin protection in sulfite sensitive asthmatics (SSA) (Abstract)." *Journal of Allergy and Clinical Immunology* (Supplement). 1984, 73:135.

**Bruce, G.** "The myth of vegetarian B12." *East West.* May 1988, pgs. 44.

**Heimburger, et al.** "Improvement in bronchial squamous metaplasia in smokers treated with folate and vitamin B12." *American Journal of Clinical Nutrition.* 1987, 45:866.

### PABA (paraaminobenzoic acid)

**Pearson, D., and Shaw, S.** *Life Extension.* 1982, pgs. 473. Warner Books, Inc. New York.

**Rosenbaum, M.E., and Bosco, D.** *Super Supplements.* 1987, pg.219.

Signet Books, New York.
**Goldstein, et al.** "PABA as a protective agent in ozone toxicity." *Archives of Environmental Health.* 1972, 24:243
**Hochschild,** "Lysosomes, membranes, and aging." *Experimental Gerontology.* 1971, 6:153.
**Kronhausen, E., and Kronhausen, P.** *Formula for Life.* 1989, p.25.William Morrow and Co. New York.
**Verzar,** "Note on the influence of Procaine, PABA, and DEAE on the aging of rats." *Gerontologia.* 1959, 3:351.

### Folic Acid (folate triglutamate)
**Heimburger, D.C., et al.** "Improvement in bronchial squamous metaplasia in smokers treated with folate and vitamin B12." *Journal of the American Medical Association.* 1988, 259:1525.
**Laurence, K.M., et al.** "Double-blind randomized controlled trial of folate treatment before conception to prevent recurrence of neural-tube defects." *British Medical Journal.* 1981, 282:1509.
**Butterworth, C.E., et al.** "Improvement of cervical dysplasia associated with folic acid therapy in users of oral contraceptives." American Journal of Clinical Nutrition. 1982, 35:73.
**Truss, C.O.** "Restoration of immunologic competence to candida albicans.". *Journal of Orthomolecular Psychiatry.* 1980, 9:287-301.
**Manzoor, M., Runcie, J.** "Folate responsive neuropathy: Report of 10 cases." *British Medical Journal.* 1976, 1:1176.
**Hillman, R.S. and Steinberg, S.E.** "The effects of alcohol on folate metabolism." *Annual Review of Medicine.* 1982, 33:345.
**Tolarova, M.** "Periconceptional supplementation with vitamins and folic acid to prevent recurrence of cleft lip." *Lancet.* 1982, 2:217.
**Rosenbaum, M.E. and Bosco, D.** *Super Supplements.* 1987, pg. 217. Signet Books, New York.
**Botez, M.I., et al.** "Neurologic disorders responsive to folic acid therapy." *Canadian Medical Association Journal.* 1976, 1:1176.
**Milunsky, A., et al.** "Multivitamin/folic acid supplementation in early pregnancy reduces the prevalence of neural tube defects." *Journal of the American Medical Association.* 1989, 262:2847.
**Smithells, R.W., et al.** "Further experience of vitamin supplementation

for prevention of neural tube defect recurrences." *Lancet.* 1983, 1:1027.
**Smithells, R.W.** "Rational use of vitamins." *Lancet.* 1984, 1:1295.

## Biotin
**Shelly, W.B. and Shelly, E.D.** "Uncombable hair syndrome: Observations on response to biotin and occurrence in siblings with ecto-dermal dysplasia." *Journal of the American Academy of Dermatology.* 1985, 13:97.
**Marshall, M.W.** "The importance of biotin-an update." *Nutrition Today.* November-December 1987, pgs. 26.
**Bonjour, J.P.** "Biotin in human nutrition." *Annals of the New York Academy of Sciences.* 1985, 447:97.
**Sydenstricker, V.P., et al.** "Observations on the "egg white injury" in man and its cure with biotin concentrate." *Journal of the American Medical Association.* 1942, 118:1199.
**Murray, M. and Pizzorno, J.** *Encyclopedia of Natural Medicine.* 1991, pgs. 284 & 504. Prima Publishing, Rocklin, Ca.

## Vitamin C
**Cathcart, R.F.** "Clinical trial of vitamin C." *Medical Tribune*, June 25, 1975.
**Cathcart, R.F.** "Vitamin C, titrating to bowel tolerance, anascorbemia, and acute induced scurvy." *Medical Hypothesis.* 1981, 7:1359.
**Cathcart, R.F.** "Vitamin C in the treatment of acquired immune defi-ciency syndrome (AIDS)." *Medical Hypothesis.* 1984, 14:423.
**Stone, I.** *The Healing Factor: Vitamin C Against Disease.* Grosset and Dunlap, New York, 1972.
**Cameron, E.** "Vitamin C." *British Journal of Hospital Medicine.* 1975, 13:511.
**Cameron, E. and Pauling, L.** "The orthomolecular treatment of cancer. I. The role of ascorbic acid in host resistance." *Chemical-Biological Interactions.* 1974, 9:273.
**Cameron, E. and Campbell, A.** "The orthomolecular treatment of can-cer. II. Clinical trial of high-dose ascorbic supplements in advanced human cancer." *Chemical-Biological Interactions.* 1974, 9:285.

163

**Cameron, E., Campbell, A. and Jack, T.** "The orthomolecular treatment of cancer. III. Reticulum cell sarcoma: double complete regression induced by high dose ascorbic acid therapy." *Chemical-Biological Interactions.* 1975, 11:387.

**Cameron, E. and Pauling, L.** "Ascorbic acid and the glycosaminoglycans: an orthomolecular approach to cancer and other diseases." *Oncology.* 1973, 27:181.

**Cameron, E. and Pauling, L.** "Supplemental ascorbate in the supportive treatment of cancer: Prolongation of survival times in terminal human cancer." Proceedings of the National Academy of Sciences USA. 1976, 73:3685.

**Cameron, E. and Pauling, L.** "Cancer and Vitamin C." 1979. Linus Pauling Institute of Science and Medicine, Palo Alto, Ca.

**Cameron, E., Pauling, L., and Leibovitz, B.** "Ascorbic acid and cancer: A Review." Cancer Research. 1979, 39:663.

**Pauling, L.** *Vitamin C and the Common Cold.* 1970. W.H. Freeman, San Francisco.

**Pauling, L.** "Evolution and the need for ascorbic acid." Proceedings of the National Academy of Sciences USA. 1970, 67:1643.

**Pauling, L.** "Preventive Nutrition." *Medicine on the Midway.* 1972, 27:15.

**Pauling, L.** "Early evidence about vitamin C and the common cold." *Journal of Orthomolecular Psychiatry.* 1974, 3:139.

**Pauling, L.** "Ascorbic acid and the common cold: Evaluation of its efficacy and toxicity." *Medical Tribune.* 1976, March 24.

**Pauling, L.** "The case for vitamin C in maintaining health and preventing disease." *Modern Medicine.* 1976, July: 68.

**Pauling, L.** *Vitamin C, the Common Cold, and the Flu.* 1976, W.H. Freeman, San Francisco.

**Rabach, J.M.** *Vitamin C for a Cold.* 1972, Dell Publishing, New York.

**Regnier, E.** "The administration of large doses of ascorbic acid in the prevention and treatment of the common cold, parts I and II." *Review of Allergy.* 1968, 22:835 and 948.

**Prinz, W., Bortz, R., Bragin, B., and Hersh, M.** "The effect of ascorbic acid supplementation on some parameters of the human immunological defense system." *International Journal of Vitamin and Nutrition Research.* 1977, 47:248.

**Anderson, R., et al.** "Ascorbic acid neutralizes reactive oxidants released by hyperactive phagocytes from cigarette smokers." *Lung.* 1988, 166:149.

**Frei, B., England, L., and Ames, B.N.** "Ascorbate is an outstanding antioxidant in human blood plasma." *Proceedings of the National Academy of Science.* 1989, 86:6377.

**Gonzales, E.R.** "Sperm swim singly after vitamin C therapy (report)." *Journal of the American Medical Association.* 1983, 249:2747.

### Vitamin E (d and or 1 tocopheryl)
**Kent, S.** "Vitamin E prevents and reverses atherosclerosis." *Life Extension Report.* 1993, 13:43.

**Grundy, S. and Jailal, I.** "Vitamin E is the best antioxidant." *Circulation.* 1993, December.

**Gonzales, E.R.** "Vitamin E relieves most cystic breast disease; may alter lipids, hormones." *Journal of the American Medical Association.* 1980, 244:1077.

**Hittner, H.M. et al.** "Retrolental fibroplasia: efficacy of Vitamin E in a double-blind clinical study of pre-term infants." *New England Journal of Medicine.* 1981, 305:1365.

**Chiswick, M.L. et al.** "Protective effect of vitamin E (dl-alpha toco-pherol) against intraventricular hemorrhage in premature babies." *British Medical Journal.* 1983, 287:81

**Steiner, M. and Anastasi, J.** "Vitamin E: An inhibitor of the platelet release reaction." *Journal of Clinical Investigations.* 1976, 57:732.

**Sobel, S. et al.** "Vitamin E in retrolental fibroplasia." (letter) *New England Journal of Medicine.* 1982, 306:867.

**Lake, A.M. et al.** "Vitamin E deficiency and enhanced platelet function. Reversal following E supplementation." *Journal of Pediatrics.* 1977, 90:722.

**Finer, N.N. et al.** "Vitamin E and necrotizing entercolitis." *Pediatrics.* 1984, 73:387.

**Weiter, J.J.** "Retrolental fibroplasia: an unsolved problem." *New England Journal of Medicine.* 1981, 305:1404.

**Chiswick, M.L. et al.** "Vitamin E and intraventricular hemorrhage in the newborn." *Annals of the New York Academy of Sciences.* 1982, 393:109.
**Farrell, P.M. and Bieri, J.G.** "Megavitamin E supplementation in man." *American Journal of Clinical Nutrition.* 1975, 28:1381.
**Bieri, J.G. et al.** "Medical uses of vitamin E." *New England Journal of Medicine.* 1983, 308:1063.
**Oski, F.A.** "Vitamin E-a radical defense." *New England Journal Of Medicine.* 1980, 303:454.
**Livingstone, P.D. and Jones, C.** "Treatment of intermittent claudication with vitamin E." *Lancet.* 1958, 2:602.
**London, R.F. et al.** "The effect of vitamin E on mammary dysplasia: A double-blind study." *Obstetrics and Gynecology.* 1985, 65:104.
**Haegar, K.** "Long-term treatment of intermittent claudication with vitamin E." American *Journal of Clinical Nutrition.* 1974, 27:1179.
**Haegar, K.** "Walking distance and arterial flow during long-term treatment of intermittent claudication with d-alpha tocopherol." *Vasa.* 1973, 2,3:280.

### Minerals
### Magnesium
**Seelig, M. and Haddy, F.** "Magnesium deficiency in arterial disease." Magnesium in Health and Disease. *Proceedings on 2nd International Symposium on Magnesium.* Montreal. 1976.
**Dyckner, T. and Wester, P.O.** "Effect of magnesium on blood pressure." *British Medical Journal.* 1983, 286:1847.
**Abraham, G.E.** "Nutritional factors in the etiology of the premenstrual tension syndromes." *Journal of Reproductive Medicine.* 1983, 28:446.
**Goei, G.S. and Abraham, G.E.** "Effect of a nutritional supplement, Optivite, a symptom of premenstrual tension." *Journal of Reproductive Medicine.* 1983, 28:527.
**Lukaski, H.C. et al.** "Maximal oxygen consumption as related to magnesium, copper, and zinc nutriture." *American Journal of Clinical Nutrition.* 1983, 37:407.
**Altura, B.M. et al.** "Magnesium deficiency and hypertension: Correlation between magnesium-deficient diets and microcirculatory

166

changes in situ." *Science.* 1984, 223:1315.

**Franz, K.B.** "Physiologic changes during a marathon with special reference to magnesium." *Journal of the American College of Nutrition.* 1985, 4:187.

**Henderson, D.G., Schierup, J. and Schodt, T.** "Effect of magnesium supplementation on blood pressure and electrolyte concentrations in hypertensive patients receiving long term diuretic treatment." *British Medical Journal.* 1986, 293:664.

**Turlapaty, P.D. and Altura, B.M.** "Magnesium deficiency produces spasms of coronary arteries: relationship to etiology of sudden death ischemic heart disease." *Science.* 1980, 208:198.

**Altura, B.M. et al.** "Magnesium deficiency-induced spasms of umbilical vessels: relation to preeclampsia, hypertension, growth retardation." *Science.* 1983, 221:376.

**Potassium**

**Khaw, K.T. and Barrett-Conner, E.** "Dietary potassium and stroke-associated mortality: A 12 year prospective population study." *New England Journal of Medicine.* 1987, 316:235.

**Khaw, K.T. and Thom, S.** "Randomized double-blind cross-over trial of potassium on blood pressure in normal subjects." *Lancet.* 1982, 2:1127.

**Schuette, S. and Linksweiler, H.** *Present Knowledge in Nutrition.* 1984. The Nutrition Foundation.

**Krishna, G.G., Miller E., and Kapoor, S.** "Increased blood pressure during potassium depletion in normotensive men." *New England Journal of Medicine.* 1989, 320:1177.

**MacGregor, G.A. et al.** "Moderate potassium supplementation in essential hypertension." *Lancet.* 1982, 2:567.

**Kronhausen, E. and Kronhausen, P.** *Formula for Life.* 1989. William Morrow and Co. New York.

**Meneely, G.R. and Battarbee, H.D.** "High sodium-low potassium environment and hypertension." *American Journal of Cardiology.* 1976, 38:768.

**Ophir, O. et al.** "Low blood pressure in vegetarians: The possible role of potassium." *American Journal of Clinical Nutrition.* 1983, 37:755.

**Skrabal, F., Aubock, J., and Hortnagl, H.** "Low sodium/high potassium diet for prevention of hypertension: Probable mechanism of action." *Lancet.* 1981, 2:895.

## Calcium
**Zaloga, G.P. and Chernow, B.** "Endocrine metabolic problems in the critically ill immunocompromised patient." In: *The Critically Ill Immunosuppressed Patient.* 1987. Aspen Publications, Inc. Rockville, Md.
**Albanese, A.A. et al.** "Calcium nutrition and skeletal and alveolar bone loss." *Nutrition Reports International.* 1985, 31:741.
**McCarron, D.A., Morris, C.D., and Cole, C.** "Dietary calcium in human hypertension." *Science.* 1982, 217:267.
**McCarron, D.A. and Morris, C.D.** "Blood pressure response to oral calcium in persons with mild to moderate hypertension." *Annals of Internal Medicine.* 1985, 103:6.
**Belizan, J.M. et al.** "Reduction of blood pressure with calcium supplementation in young adults." *Journal of the American Medical Association.* 1983, 249:1161.
**Appleton, G.V.N. et al.** "Inhibition of intestinal carcinogenesis by dietary supplementation with calcium." *British Journal of Surgery.* 1987, 74:523.
**Belizan, J.M. et al.** Preliminary evidence of the effect of calcium supplementation on blood pressure in normal pregnant women." *American Journal of Obstetrics and Gynecology.* 1983, 146:175.

## Vitamin D3 (cholecalciferol)
**Thompson, D.S.** *Every Woman's Health.* 1993, p.68. Simon and Schuster, New York.
**Parfitt, A.M. et al.** "Vitamin D and bone health in the elderly." *American Journal of Clinical Nutrition.*" 1982, 36:1014.
**Crowle, A.J., Ross, E.J., and May, M.H.** "Inhibition by 1,25(0H)2vitamin D3 of the multiplication of virulent tubercle bacilli in cultured human macrophages." *Infection and Immunity* 1987, 55:2945.
**Harju, E. et al.** "High incidence of low serum vitamin D concentration in patients with hip fracture." *Archives of Orthopedic and Traumatic*

*Surgery.* 1985, 103:408.

**Garland, C. et al.** "Dietary vitamin D and calcium and risk of colorectal cancer: A 19 year prospective study in men." *Lancet.* 1985, 1:307.

**Selenium (sodium selenate and seleno+methionine-Nutr. 21)**

**Yu, S.Y. et al.** "Regional variation of cancer mortality incidence and its relation to selenium levels in China." *Biological Trace Element Research.* 1985, 7:21.

**Shamberger, R.J. et al.** "Antioxidants and cancer. Part VI. Selenium and age-adjusted human cancer mortality." *Archives of Environmental Health.* 1976, 31:231.

**Shamberger, R.J.** "Relationship of selenium to cancer: I. Inhibitory effect of selenium on carcinogenesis." *Journal of the National Cancer Institute.* 1970, 44:931.

**Dworkin, B.M. et al.** "Selenium deficiency in the acquired immunodeficiency syndrome." *Journal of Parenteral and Enteral Nutrition.* 1986, 10:405.

**Salonen, J.T. et al.** "Risk of cancer in relation to serum concentrations of selenium and vitamins A and E: matched case control analysis of prospective data." *British Medical Journal.* 1985, 290:417.

**Perry, H.M. Jr. and Erlanger, M.W.** "Prevention of cadmium-induced hypertension by selenium." *Federal Proceedings.* 1974, 33:357.

**Schrauzer, G.N. et al.** "Cancer mortality correlation studies. Part III. Statistical associations with dietary selenium intakes." *Bioinorganic Chemistry.* 1977, 7:23.

**Schrauzer, G.N. et al.** "Selenium in human nutrition-dietary intakes and effects of supplementation." *Bioinorganic Chemistry.* 1978, 8:303.

**Mondragon, M.C. and Jaffe, W.G.** "The ingestion of selenium in Caracas compared with some other cities of the world." *Archives of Latinoamerican Nutrition.* 1976, 26:341.

**Greeder, G.A. and Milner J.A.** "Factors influencing the inhibitory effect of selenium on mice inoculated with Ehrlich ascites tumor cells." *Science.* 1980:209.

**Yang, G. et al.** "Endemic selenium intoxication of humans in China." *American Journal of Clinical Nutrition.* 1983, 37:872.

**Thompson, H.J. and Becci, P.J.** "Selenium inhibition of N-methyl, N-nitrosourea-induced mammary carcinogenesis in the rat." *Journal of the National Cancer Institute.* 1980, 65:1299.

**Hendler, S.S.** *The Doctors Vitamin and Mineral Encyclopedia.* Simon and Schuster, New York. 1990, p.185

## Amino Acids.
### L-Taurine

**Hayes, K.C., Carey, R.E., and Schmidt, S.Y.** "Retinal degeneration associated with taurine deficiency in the cat." *Science.* 1975, 188:949.

**Chaitow, L.** *Thorsons Guide to Amino Acids.* HarperCollins, London. 1991, p.68.

**Takihara, K. et al.** "Beneficial effect of taurine in rabbits with chronic congestive heart failure." *American Heart Journal.* 1986, 112:1278.

**Azuma, J. et al.** "Therapeutic effect of taurine in congestive heart failure: A double-blind crossover trial." *Clinical Cardiology.* 1985, 8:276.

**Rosenbaum, M.E. and Bosco, D.** *Super Supplements.* 1987. Signet Books New York.

**Pion, P.D.** "Miocardial failure in cats associated with low plasma taurine: A reversible cardiomyopathy." *Science.* 1987, 237:764.

**Belli, D.C. et al.** "Taurine improves the absorption of a fat meal in patients with cystic fibrosis." *Pediatrics.* 1987, 80:517.

**Barbeau, A.** "Zinc, taurine and epilepsy." *Archives of Neurology.* 1974, 30:52.

**Barbeau, A.** "The neuropharmacology of taurine." *Life Sciences.* 1975, 17:669.

### N-Acetyl-Cysteine

**Anderson, R., Theron, A.J., and Ras, G.J.** "Regulation by the antioxidants ascorbate, cysteine, and dapsone of the increased extracellular and intracellular generation of reactive oxidants by activated phagocytes from cigarette smokers." *American Review of Respiratory Diseases.* 1987, 135:1027.

**Pearson, D. and Shaw, S.** *Life Extension.* Warner Books, New York. 1982, p. 267.

**Pearson, D. and Shaw, S.** "Cysteine-the sulfur connection." *Anti-Aging News.* 1982, 2:5.

**Forman, H.J., Rotman, E.I., and Fisher, A.B.** "Role of selenium and sulfur containing amino acids in protection against oxygen toxicity." *Laboratory Investigation.* 1983, 49:148.

**Oeriu, S., and Vochitu, E.** "The effect of the administration of compounds which contain sulfhydril groups on the survival rates of mice, rats, and guinea pigs." *Journal of Gerontology.* 1965, 20:417.

**Springe, et al.** "Protectants against acetaldehyde toxicity: Sulfhydryl compounds and ascorbic acid." Federal Proceedings. *Federation of the American Society for Experimental Biology.* 1974, 172:233.

### Cholinergenic Complex
### Choline bitartrate and phosphatidyl choline

**Kosina, F. et al.** "Essential cholinephospholipids in the treatment of virus hepatitis (translated from Czech)." *Casopis Lekaru Ceskych.* 1981, 120.

**Atoba, M.A., Ayoola, E.A., and Ogunseyinde, O.** "Effect of essential phospholipid choline on the course of acute hepatitis-B infection." *Tropical Gastroenterology.* 1985, 6(2):96.

**Visco, G.** "Polyunsaturated phosphatidylcholine in association with vitamin B complex in the treatment of acute viral hepatitis B (translated from Italian)." *Clinical Terapeutica.* 1985, 114:183.

**Kent, S.** *Your Personal Life Extension Program.* 1985, p.154. William Morrow and Co.

**Cohen, B.M., Lipinski, J.F., and Altesman, R.I.** "Lecithin in the treatment of mania: Double-blind, placebo controlled trials." *American Journal of Psychiatry.* 1982, 139:1162.

**Jackson, I.V. et al.** "Treatment of tardive dyskinesia with lecithin." *American Journal of Psychiatry.* 1979, 136:1458.

**Gelenberg, A.J., Doller-Wojcik, J.C. and Growden, J.H.** "Choline and lecithin in the treatment of tardive dyskinesia: Preliminary results from a pilot study." *American Journal of Psychiatry.* 1979, 136:772.

**Hendler, S.S.** *The Doctors Vitamin and Mineral Encyclopedia.* 1990, p.261. Simon and Schuster, New York.

**Jenkins, P.J. et al.** "Use of polyunsaturated phosphatidyl choline in

171

HBsAg negative chronic active hepatitis: Results of prospective double-blind controlled trial." *Liver.* 1982, 2:77.

**Growden, J.H. et al.** "Lecithin can suppress tardive dyskinesia." *New England Journal of Medicine.*" 1978, 298:1029.

**Growden, J.H. et al.** "Oral choline administration to patients with tardive dyskinesia." *New England Journal of Medicine.* 1977, 297:524.

## Inositol

**Clements, R.S., Jr. et al.** "Dietary myo-inositol intake and peripheral nerve function in diabetic neuropathy." *Metabolism.* 1979, 28:477.

**Pearson, D. and Shaw, S.** *Life Extension.* Warner Books, New York. 1982, p.476.

**Gregersen, G. et al.** "Oral supplementation of myo-inositol: Effects on peripheral nerve function in human diabetics and concentration in plasma, erythrocytes, urine and muscle tissue in human diabetics and normals." *Acta Neurologica Scandinavica.* 1983, 67:164.

## Flavonoid Complex

**Middleton, E.J.** "The flavonoids." *Trends in Pharmacological Sciences.* 1984, 8:335.

**Middleton, E.J., Drzewiecki, G., and Tatum, J.** "The effects of citrus flavonoids on human basophil and neutrophil function." *Planta Medica.* 1987, 53:325.

**Null, G.** *No More Allergies.* 1992, p.298. Villard Books, New York.

**Havsteen, B.** "Flavonoids, a class of natural products of high pharmacological potency." *Biochemical Pharmacology.* 1983, 32:1141.

**Kaul, T.N., Middleton, E., and Ogra, P.L.** "Antiviral effect of flavonoids on human viruses." *Journal of Medical Virology.* 1985, 15:71.

**Spedding, G., Ratty, A., and Middleton, E.J.** "Inhibition of reverse transcriptases by flavonoids." *Antiviral Research.* 1989, 12:99.

## Additional nutrients.
### Dilaurylthiodipropionate and thiodipropionic acid.

**Pearson, D. and Shaw, S.** *Life Extension.* 1982, p.476 & 381. Warner books, New York.

## Bromelain

**Rosenbaum, M. and Bosco, D.** *Super Supplements.* 1987, p.106 & 236. Signet books, New York.

**Pearson, D. and Shaw, S.** *Life Extension.* 1982. p.237. Warner Books, New York.

**Murray, M. and Pizzorno, J.** *Encyclopedia of Natural Medicine.* 1991, p. 513. Prima Publishing, Rocklin, Ca.

**Taussig, S., Yokoyama, M., Chinen, A. et al.** "Bromelain, a proteolytic enzyme and its clinical application: A review." *Hiroshima Journal of Medical Science.* 1975, 24:185.

**Taussig, S.** "The mechanism of the physiological action of bromelain." *Medical Hypothesis.* 1960, 6:99.

## Additional minerals
## Zinc.

**Brewer, G.J. et al.** "Oral zinc therapy for Wilson's disease." *Annals of Internal Medicine.* 1983, 99:314.

**Fell, G.S.** "The link with zinc." *British Medical Journal.* 1985, 290:242.

**Michaelsson, G.** "Oral zinc in acne." *Acta Dermatovener* (supplement). 1980, 89:87.

**Anonymous.** "Oral zinc therapy for Wilson's disease." *Nutrition Review.* 1984, 42:184.

**Schachner, L.** "The treatment of acne: A contemporary review." *Pediatric Clinics of North America.* 1983, 30:501.

**Reding, P. et al.** "Oral zinc supplementation improves hepatic encephalopathy. Results of a randomized controlled trial." *Lancet.* 1984, 2:493.

**Myers, M.B. and Cherry, G.** "Zinc and the healing of chronic leg ulcers." *American Journal of Surgery.* 1970, 120:77.

**Mukherjee, M.D. et al.** "Maternal zinc, iron, folic acid, and protein nutriture and outcome of human pregnancy." *American Journal of Clinical Nutrition.* 1984, 40:496.

**Pories, W.J. et al.** "Acceleration of wound healing in man with zinc sulphate given by mouth." *Lancet.* 1969, 1:1069.

**Hunt, I.F. et al.** "Zinc supplemental during pregnancy: Effects on selected blood constituents and on progress and outcome of pregnancy in low income women of Mexican descent." *American Journal of Clinical Nutrition.* 1984, 40:508.

**Fraker, P.J. et al.** "Interrelationships between zinc and immune function." *Federal Proceedings.* 1986, 45:1479.

**Hoogenraad, T.U. et al.** "Effect treatment of Wilson's disease with oral zinc sulfate: Two case reports." *British Medical Journal.* 1984, 289:273.

**Frommer, D.J.** "The healing of gastric ulcers by zinc sulfate." *Medical Journal of Australia.* 1975, 2:793.

**Tuttle, S. et al.** "Zinc and copper in human pregnancy: A longitudinal study in normal primigravidae and in primigravidae at risk of delivering a growth retarded baby." *American Journal of Clinical Nutrition.* 1985, 41:1032.

**Kinlaw, W.B. et al.** "Abnormal zinc metabolism in type II diabetes mellitus." *American Journal of Medicine.* 1983, 75:273.

**Hendler S.S.** *The Doctors Vitamin and Mineral Encyclopedia.* 1990, p.202. Simon and Schuster, New York.

### ChromeMate GTF and chromium picolinate

**Offenbacher, E.G. and Pi-Sunyer, F.X.** "Beneficial effect of chromium-rich yeast on glucose tolerance and blood lipids in elderly subjects." *Diabetes.* 1980, 29:919.

**Offenbacher, E.G. and Pi-Sunyer, F.X.** "Chromium in human nutrition." *Annual Review of Nutrition.* 1988, 8:543.

**Liu, V.J.K. et al.** "Effects of high-chromium yeast-extract supplementation on serum lipids, serum insulin, and glucose tolerance in older women." *Federal Proceedings.* 1977, 36:1123.

**Liu, V.J.K. and Morris, J.S.** "Relative chromium response as an indicator of chromium status." *American Journal of Clinical Nutrition.* 1978, 31:972.

**Abraham, A.S. et al.** "The effect of chromium on established atherosclerotic plaques in rabbits." *American Journal of Clinical Nutrition.* 1980, 33:2294.

**Glinsmann, W.H. and Mertz, W.** "Effect of trivalent chromium on glucose tolerance." *Metabolism.* 1966, 15:510.

**Press, R.I., Geller, J., and Evans, G.W.** "The effect of chromium picolinate on serum cholesterol and apolipoprotein fractions in human subjects." *Western Journal of Medicine.* 1990, 152:41.

**Martinez, O.B.** "Dietary chromium and effect of chromium supplementation on glucose tolerance of elderly Canadian women." *Nutrition Research.* 1985, 5:609.

**Mertz, W.** "Effects and metabolism of glucose tolerance factor." *Nutrition Review.* 1975, 33:129.

**Canfield, W.** "Chromium, glucose tolerance, and cholesterol in adults." In: Shapcott, D. and Hubert, J. (eds.). *Chromium in Nutrition and Metabolism.* Amsterdam: Elsevier. 1979, p.145.

**Potter, J.F. et al.** "Glucose metabolism in glucose intolerant older people during chromium supplementation." *Metabolism.* 1985. 34:199.

**Anderson, R.A. et al.** "Chromium supplementation of humans with hypoglycemia." *Federation Proceedings.* 1984, 43:471.

**Mossop, R.T.** "Effects of chromium III on fasting blood glucose, cholesterol, and cholesterol HDL levels in diabetics." *Central African Journal of Medicine.* 1983, 29:80.

**Anderson, R.A. et al.** "Effects of supplemental chromium on patients with symptoms of reactive hypoglycemia." *Metabolism.* 1987, 35:351.

**Kovlovsky, A.S. et al.** "Effects of diets high in simple sugars on urinary chromium losses." *Metabolism.* 1986, 35:515.

**Bunker, W. et al.** "The uptake and excretion of chromium by the elderly." *American Journal of Clinical Nutrition.* 1984, 39:799.

**Elias, A.N., Grossman, M.K., and Valenta, L.J.** "Use of the artificial beta cell (ABC) in the assessment of peripheral insulin sensitivity: Effect of chromium supplementation in diabetics." *General Pharmacology.* 1984, 15:535.

## Molybdenum

**Null, G.** *No More Allergies.* 1992, p.82. Villard books, New York.

**Rajagopalan, K.V.** "Molybdenum: An essential trace element." *Nutrition Review.* 1987, 45(11):321.

Rajagopalan, K.V. "Molybdenum: An essential trace element in human nutrition." *Annual Review of Nutrition*. 1988, 8:401.

**Coordinating Group for Research on Etiology of Esophageal Cancer in North China.** "The epidemiology and etiology of esophageal cancer in North China." *Chinese Medical Journal*. 1975, 1(3):167.

Luo, X.M. et al. "Molybdenum and esophageal cancer in China." *Federation Proceedings*. Federation of the American Society for Experimental Biology. 1981, 46:928.

Hendler, S.S. *The Doctors' Vitamin and Mineral Encyclopedia*. 1990, p.170. Simon and Schuster, New York.

### Manganese

Null, G. *No More Allergies*. 1992, p.11 & 50. Villard books, New York.

Hendler, S.S. *The Doctors' Vitamin and Mineral Encyclopedia*. 1990, p.167.

Pfeiffer, C.C. *Zinc and Other Micro-Nutrients*. 1978, p.66. Keats publishing, New Canaan, Conn.

Freeland-Graves, J.H. "Manganese: An essential nutrient for humans." *Nutrition Today*. 1988, p.13, Nov.-Dec.

Friedman, B.J. et al. "Manganese balance and clinical observations in young men fed a manganese deficient diet." *Journal of Nutrition*. 1987, 117:133.

### Iodine

Hamner, D. and Burr, B. *Peak Energy*. 1988, p.124. G.P. Putnam's Sons, New York.

Becker, D.V. et al. "The use of iodine as a thyroidal blocking agent in the event of a reactor accident." *Journal of the American Medical Association*. 1984, 252:659.

Anonymous. "Iodine relieves pain of fibrocystic breasts"(Report). *Medical World News*. 1988, p.25, Jan.11.

### Phenylalanine

"Phenylalanine: A psychoactive nutrient for some depressives?" *Medical World News*. October 27, 1983.

176

**Beckman, H.** "Phenylalanine in affective disorders." *Advanced Biological Psychiatry.* 1983, 10:137.

**Beckman, H. et al.** "DL-phenylananine versus imipramine: A double-blind controlled study." *Archiv fur Psychiatrie und Nervenkrankheiten.* 1979, 227:49.

**Beckman, VH. and Ludolph, E.** "DL-phenylalanine as antidepressant." *Arzneimittel-Forschung.* 1978, 28:1283.

**Budd, K.** "Use of D-phenylalanine, an enkephalinase inhibitor, in the treatment of intractable pain." *Advances in Pain Research and Therapy.* 1983, 5:305.

**Ehrenpreis, S. et al.** Further studies on the analgesic activity of D-phenylananine (DPA) in mice and humans. In: Way, EL (ed.), *Endogenous and Exogenous Opiate Agonists and Antagonists.* New York , Pergamon Press, 1980, p.379.

**Hyodo, M., Kitada, T., and Hosoka, E.** "Study on the enhanced analgesic effect induced by phenylananine during acupuncture analgesia in humans." *Advances in Pain Research and Therapy.* 1983, 5:577.

**Kravitz, HM., Sabelli, HC., and Fawcett, J.** "Dietary supplements of phenylananine and other amino acid precursors of brain neuroamines in the treatment of depressive disorders." *Journal of the American Osteopathic Association.* 1984, 84:119.

### Creatine

**Sipila, I., et al.** "Supplementary creatine as a treatment for gyrate atrophy of the choroid and retina". *New England Journal of Medicine,* 1981, 304;867.

**Loike, J.D. et al.** "Extracellular creatine regulates creatine transport in rat and human cells". *Proceedings of the National Academy of Sciences,* 1988, 85;807.

**Harris, R.C. et al.** "Evaluation of creatine in resting and exercised muscle of normal subjects by creatine supplementation". *Clinical Science,* 1992, 83;367.

**Guimbal, C., and Kilimann, M.W.** "A Na+-dependent creatine transporter in rabbit brain, muscle, heart, and kidney". *The Journal of Biological Chemistry,* 1993, 268;8416.

**Greenhaff, P.L. et al** "Influence of oral creatine supplementation of muscle torque during repeated bouts of maximal voluntary exercise in man". *Clinical Science*, 1993, 84;565.
**Almada, A.** "The creatine muscle growth mystique and the (possible) IGF-1 or clenbuterol connection". *Muscle Media 2000*, Jan.1995, 41;31.

### Ornithine alpha-ketoglutarate (OKG)
**LeBricon, T; Cynober, L; Baracos, VE.** "Ornithine alpha-ketoglutarate limits muscle protein breakdown without stimulating tumor growth in rats bearing yoshida ascites hepatoma." *Metabolism*, 1994, 43:899.
**Braverman, ER. Pfieffer, CC.** eds. *The Healing Nutrients Within Facts, Findings, and New Research on Amino Acids.* 1986, p.106. New Cannan: Keats.
**Cynobar, L. et al.** "Action of ornithine alpha-ketoglutarate on protein metabolism in burn patients." *Nutrition.* 1987, 3:187.
**Cynobar, L. et al.** "Action of ornithine alpha-ketoglutarate, ornithine hydrochloride, and calcium alpha-ketoglutarate on plasma amino acid and hormonal patterns in healthy subjects." *Journal of the American College of Nutrition.* 1990, 9:2.
**Crist, DM. et al.** "Body composition response to exogenous growth hormone during training in highly conditioned athletes." *Journal of Applied Physiology.* 1988, 65:579.
**Wernerman J. et al.** "Ornithine alpha-ketoglutarate improves skeletal muscle protein synthesis as assessed by ribosome analysis and nitrogen balance postoperatively." *Annals of Surgery.* 1987, 206:674.
**Vaubourdolle, M. et al.** "Action of enterally administered ornathine alpha-ketoglutarate on protein breakdown in skeletal muscle and liver of the burned rat." *Journal of Parenteral and Enteral Nutrition.* 1991, 15:517.
**Leander, U. et al.** "Nitrogen sparing effects of ornithine in the immediate post operative state." *Clinical Nutrition.* 1985, 4:43.

### Protein
**Millward, DJ, Rivers HPW,** "The need for indispensable amino acids: The concept of the anabolic drive." *Diabetes Melab Review*, 1989, 5:191.

*Recommended Dietary Allowances,* 10th Edition. Washington, D.C. 1989, National Academy Press.

**McCarthy, P.** "How much protein do athletes really need?" *The Physician and Sports Medicine.* May, 1989. 17:5, 170.

**Lemon, P. Mullin, J.** "Effect of initial muscle glycogen levels on protein catabolism during exercise". *Journal of Applied Physiology.* 1980, 48:624.

**Lemon, P.** "Protein and exercise: Update 1987." *Medicine and Science in Sports and Exercise.* 1987, 19:S179.

**Colgan, M., Fielder, MS. Colgan, LA.** "Micronutrient status of endurance athletes affects hematology and performance." *Journal of Applied Nutrition.* 1991, 43:17.

**Colgan, M.** *Optimum Sports Nutrition.* 1993, Advanced Research Press. 142-165.

**Gontzea, I. Sutzescu, P. Dumitrache, S.** "The influence of muscular activity on nitrogen balance and on the need of man for proteins." *Nutrition Reports International.* 1974, 10:35.

**Gontzea, I. Sutzesca, R. Dumitrache, S.** "The influence of adaptation to physical effort on nitrogen balance in man." *Nutrition Reports International.* 1975, 11:231.

"How Much Protein Do Athletes Really Need?" *Tufts University Diet and Nutrition Letter*, 1987, 5:1.

**Passwater, R.** *Supernutrition.* 1975, Dial Press, New York.

### Anti-alcohol antioxidants.
**Anderson, R., Theron, A.J., and Ras, G.J.** "Regulation by the antioxidants ascorbate, cysteine, and dapsone of the increased extracellular and intracellular generation of reactive oxidants by activated phagocytes from cigarette smokers." *American Review of Respiratory Diseases.* 1987, 135:1027.

**Pearson, D. and Shaw, S.** *Life Extension.* Warner Books, New York. 1982, p. 267.

**Pearson, D. and Shaw, S.** "Cysteine-the sulfur connection." *Anti-Aging News.* 1982, 2:5.

**Forman, H.J., Rotman, E.I., and Fisher, A.B.** "Role of selenium and

179

sulfur containing amino acids in protection against oxygen toxicity." *Laboratory Investigation.* 1983, 49:148.

**Oeriu, S., and Vochitu, E.** "The effect of the administration of compounds which contain sulfhydril groups on the survival rates of mice, rats, and guinea pigs." *Journal of Gerontology.* 1965, 20:417.

**Springe, et al.** "Protectants against acetaldehyde toxicity: Sulfhydryl compounds and ascorbic acid." *Federal Proceedings.* Federation of the American Society for Experimental Biology. 1974, 172:233.

**Sprince, et al.** "L-ascorbic acid in alcoholism and smoking: Protection against acetaldehyde toxicity as an experimental model." *International Journal for Vitamin and Nutrition Research.* 1977, 47:185.

### Cranberry extract

**Prodromos, P., Brusch, C., and Ceresia, G.** "Cranberry juice in the treatment of urinary tract infections." Southwest Medicine. 1968, 47:17.

**Sternlieb, P.** "Cranberry juice in renal disease." *New England Journal of Medicine.* 1963, 268:57

**Bodel, P., Cotran, R., and Kass, E.** Cranberry juice and the antibacterial action of hippuric acid." *Journal of Laboratory and Clinical Medicine.* 1959, 54:881.

**Moen, D.** "Observations on the effectiveness of cranberry juice in urinary infections." *Wisconsin Medical Journal.* 1962, 61:282.

### Garlic

**Norwell, D. and Tarr, R.** "Garlic, vampires, and coronary heart disease." *Osteopathic Annals.* 1984, 12:276.

**Bordia, A., Josh, H., and Sanadhya, Y.** "Effect of garlic oil on fibrinolytic activity in patient with coronary heart disease." *Atherosclerosis.* 1977, 28:155.

**Block, E.** "The chemistry of garlic and onions." *Scientific American.* 1985, 252:114.

**Harris, L.** *The Book of Garlic.* 1979. Aris Books, Harris Publishing Co.

**Kendler, B.** "Garlic (allium sativum) and onion(allium cepa): A review of their relationship to cardiovascular disease." *Preventive Medicine.* 1987, 16:670.

**Weber, N. et al.** "Antiviral activity of allium sativum (garlic)." *88th meeting of The American Society for Microbiology. Abstract A-126.* 1988, p. 22.

## Flaxseed Oil—EPA/DHA

**Allen, B., et al.** "The effects on psoriasis of dietary supplementation with eicosapentaenoic acid." *British Journal of Dermatology.* 1986, 113:777.

**Friday, K., et al.** "The effect of omega-3 fatty acid supplementation on glucose homeostasis and plasma lipoproteins in type II diabetic subjects." *American Journal of Clinical Nutrition.* 1987, 45:871.

**Chandra, R.** "There is more to fish than fish oils." *Nutrition Research.* 1988, 8:1.

**Dyerberg, J.** "Linolenate-derived polyunsaturated fatty acids and prevention of atherosclerosis." *Nutrition Reviews.* 1986, 44:125.

**Sanders, T. and Roshanai, F.** "The influence of different types of omega-3 polyunsaturated fatty acidson blood lipids sand platelet function in healthy volunteers." *Clinical Science.* 1983, 64:91.

**Renaud, S. and Norday, A.** "Small is beautiful: alpha-linolenic acid and eicosapentaenoic acid in man." *Lancet.* 1983, i, p.1,169.

**Glauber, H., et al.** "Adverse effect of omega-3 fatty acids in non-insulin dependent diabetes mellitus." *Annals of Internal Medicine.* 1988, 108:663.

**Anderson, G. and Conner, W.** "On the demonstration of omega-3 essential fatty acid deficiency in humans." (editorial) *American Journal of Clinical Nutrition.* 1989, 49:585.

**Conner, W., Harris, W., and Rothrock, D., et al.** "Reduction of plasma lipids, lipoproteins, and apoproteins by dietary fish oils in patients with hypertriglyceridemia." *New England of Medicine.* 1985, 312:1,210.

**Holman, R., Johnson, S., and Hatch, T.** "A case of human linolenic acid deficiency involving neurological abnormalities." *American Journal of Clinical Nutrition.* 1982, 65:617.

**Catherine, E. et al.** "Topical eicosapentaenoic acid (EPA) in the treatment of psoriasis." *British Journal of Dermatology.* 1989, 120:581.

## Nasturtium

**Duke, J.** *Handbook of Medicinal Herbs.* 1985, CRC Press, Boca Raton, Fla.

**Elden, ed.** *Biophysical Properties of the Skin.* 1971, Wiley Interscience.

**Wagner, H.,** "Plant constituents with antihepatotoxic activity," in Beal J. and Richard, E., (eds.) *Natural Products as Medicinal Agents,* Hippokrates-Verlag, Stuttgart, 1981.

**Rao, C. Rao, V., and Steinman, B.** "Influence of bioflavonoids on the metabolism and crosslinking of collagen." *Italian Journal of Biochemistry.* 1981, 30, p.259.

**Verzar.** "The aging of collagen." *Scientific American.* April 1963.

*Life Extension Update.* 1995, April 5, p.3.

**Leung, A.** *Encyclopedia of Common Natural Ingredients Used in Food, Drugs, and Cosmetics.* 1980. John Wiley and Sons. New York.

## Rejuvenex

**Laden and Spitzer.** "Identification of a natural moisturizing agent in skin." *Journal of the Society of Cosmetic Chemists.* 1967,18:351.

**Goldfarb, M.T., et al.** "Topical tretinoin therapy: its use in photoaged skin." *Journal of the American Academy of Dermatology.* 1989, 645.

**Schachner, L.** "The treatment of acne: A contemporary review." *Pediatric Clinics of North America.* 1983, 30:501.

**Forman, H.J., Rotman, E.I., and Fisher, A.B.** "Role of selenium and sulfur containing amino acids in protection against oxygen toxicity." *Laboratory Investigation.* 1983, 49:148.

*The Salts of PCA and their Moisturizing Effects.* Technical Bulletin, Ajinomoto Company (8 references).

## N-Zimes

**Innerfield, I.** Enzymes in Clinical Medicine. 1960, McGraw Hill, New York.

**Steffen, C., and Menzel, J.** In vivo breakdown of immune complexes in the kidney by oral administration of enzymes." *Wiener Klinische Wochenschrift.* 1987, 99:525.

**Pearson, D. and Shaw, S.** *Life Extension.* 1983. Warner Books, New York.

# BioPro

**Will, T.** "Lactobacillus overgrowth for treatment of monilary vulvo-vaginitis," (letter). *Lancet.* 1979, 2:482.

**Anderson, K., Anderson, L. and Glanze, W. eds.** *Mosby's Medical Dictionary.* 1994, 4th edition, Mosby Yearbook, Inc. St. Louis Missouri. Health and Longevity: The probiotic revolution. *Health/Science Newsletter,* special issue, 1995.

**Friend, B., et al.** "Nutritional and therapeutic aspects of lactobacilli." *Journal of Applied Nutrition.* 1984,36:125.

**Gotz, V. et al.** "Prophylaxis against ampicillin-associated diarrhea with lactobacillus preparation." *American Hospital Pharmacy.* 1979, 36:754.

# CHAPTERS 22-24

**Pearson, D. and Shaw, S.** *Life Extension.* 1983, pgs. 115, 306, 390, 485 . Warner Books, New York.

**Kronhausen, E. and Kronhausen, P.** *Formula For Life.* 1989, pgs.22, 41, 70 and 73. William Morrow, New York.

**Arfors, K.,** Chairman, Pharmacia Symposium #1. "Free radicals in medicine and biology." *Acta Phsiologica Scandinavica.* 1980, (supplement 492) 492:1.

**Bendich, A., Machlin, l., Scandurra, O., Burton, G., and Wayner D.** "The antioxidant role of vitamin C." *Advances in Free Radical Biology and Medicine.* 1986, 2:419.

**Bulkley, G.** "The role of oxygen free radicals in human disease processes." *Surgery.* 1983, 94:407.

**Burton, G. and Ingold, K.** "Beta carotene: An unusual type of lipid antioxidant." *Science.* 1984, 224:569.

**Demopoulos, H.** "Control of free radicals in the biologic systems." *Federal Proceedings.* 1973, 32:1903.

**Demopolous, H.** "The basis of free radical pathology." *Ibid.,* 1973, 1859.

**Dormandy, T.** "Free radicals and alcoholism" (letter). *Lancet.* 1985, 956.

**Dormandy, T.** "Free radical oxidation and antioxidants." *Lancet.* 1978, 647.

**Pauling, L.** *How To Live Longer and Feel Better.* 1986, p.166. W.H.

Freeman and Co. New York.

**Harman, D.** "Free radical theory of aging: Nutritional implications." *Age.* 1978, 1(4): 145.

**Harman, H.** "Free radical theory of aging." *Journal of Gerontology.* 1968, 23(4).

*Pesticides in Food.* Hearings of the Subcommittee on Oversight and Investigations of the Committee on Energy and Commerce, 100th Congress, 1st session. 1987, April 30.

**McKenna, A, et al.** *Pesticide Regulation Handbook.* Washington, DC. 1987.

*Americas Pest Control Predicament.* Washington, DC. Public Citizen. 1987.

**Harris, R. Karmas, E. eds.** *Nutritional Evaluation of Food Processing,* 2nd edition. 1975. Avi Publishing, Westport, Connecticut.

**Colgan, M.** *The New Nutrition.* 1994, p.10. CI Publications, Encinitas, Ca.

**Pottenger, F.** "The effects of heated, processed foods and vitamin D milk on the dental facial structure of experimental animals." *American Journal of Orthodontics and Oral Surgery.* August, 1946.

**Pike, M. et al.** "Age at onset of lung cancer: Significance in relation to effect of smoking." *Lancet.* 1965, March.

**Bauernfeind, J.** *Food Sources of the Tocopherols. In Vitamin E: A Comprehensive Treatise.* 1980, pg. 104

**Willner, R.,** *The Cancer Solution.* 1994, p. 224. Peltec Publishing, Boca Raton, Fla.

**McTaggart, L.** *Medical Madness.* 1995, p.70. What Doctors Don't Tell You (publishers). Baltimore, Md.

**Wolfe, S. M.** *13,012 Questionable Doctors.* 1996.

**Wolfe, S.M. and Hope, R.** *Worst Pills Best Pills II.* 1993, Public Citizen Health Research Group.

## SECTION III

**Cooper, KH.** *Aerobics.* 1968, Bantam Books, New York.

**Blair, SN., Kohl, HW., Gordon, NF., and Paffenbarger, RS, Jr.** "How

184

much physical activity is good for health?" *Annual Review of Public Health* (US), 1992, 13:99.

**Blair, SN., Kohl, HW., Barlow, CE., et al.** "Changes in physical fitness and all-cause mortality." *Journal of the American Medical Association.* 1995, 273:1093.

**Sherman, SE., D'Agostino, RB., Cobb, JL., and Kannel, WB.** "Does exercise reduce mortality rates in the elderly? Experience from the framingham heart study." *American Heart Journal* (US), Nov., 1994, 128 (5):965.

**Sherman, SE., D'Agostino, RB., Cobb, JL., and Kannel, WB.** "Physical activity and mortality in women in the framingham heart study." *American Heart Journal* (US), Nov. 1994, 128 (5):879.

**Paffenbarger, RS Jr., Hyde, RT., Wing AL., et al.** "The association of changes in physical-activity level and other lifestyle characteristics with mortality among men." *New England Journal of Medicine.* 1993, 328:538.

**Paffenbarger, RS Jr., Kampert, JB., Lee, IM., et al.** "Changes in physical activity and other lifeway patterns influencing longevity." *Medicine and Science in Sports and Exercise.* 1994, 26:857.

**Paffenbarger, RS, Jr., Hyde, RT., Wing, AL., and Hsieh, CC.** "Physical activity, all-cause mortality and longevity of college alumni." *New England Journal of Medicine* (US), Mar 6, 1986, 314 (10):605.

**Lee, IM., Hsieh, CC., and Paffenbarger, RS, Jr.** "Exercise intensity and longevity in men - the Harvard alumni health study." *Journal of American Medical Association* (US), Apr. 19, 1995, 273 (15):1179.

**Sarna, S., Shai, T., Koskenvuo, M., and Kaprio, J.** "Increased life expectancy of world class male athletes." *Medicine and Science in Sports and Exercise* (US), Feb., 1993, 25 (2):237.

**Berger, RA.** "Optimum repetitions for the development of strength." *Research Quarterly*, 1962, 33:334.

**Elliott, BC., Wilson, GJ., and Kerr, GK.** " A biomechanical analysis of the sticking region in the bench press." *Medicine and Science in Sports and Exercise*, 1989, 21:450.

**Fleck, SJ and Kraemer, WJ.** *Designing Resistance Training Program.* Human Kinetics Publishing, 1987.

**Newton, RU., and Wilson, GJ.** "Reducing the risk of injury during plyometric training: The effect of dampeners." *Sports Medicine, Training and Rehabilitation,* 1993 4:1.

**Young,WB.** "Training for speed/strength: Heavy versus light loads." *NSCA,* 1993, 15 (5):34.

**Young, WB and Bilby, GE.** "The effect of voluntary effort to influence speed of contraction on strength, muscular power and hypertrophy development." *Journal of Strength and Conditioning Research,* 1993, 7 (3):172.

**Parkhouse, WS., Willis, PE., and Zhang, J.** "Hepatic lipid peroxidation and antioxidant enzyme responses to long-term voluntary physical activity and aging." *Age Journal,* 1995, 18:11.

**Erikssen, J.** "Physical fitness and coronary heart disease morbidity and mortality: A prospective study in apparently healthy, middle-aged men." *Acta Medical Scandinavica* Supplement. 1986, 711:189

**Kraemer, WJ.,**"Endocrine responses and adaptations to strength training." *The Encyclopedia of Sports Medicine: Strength and Power.* Blackwell Scientific Publishing, Oxford, 1992.

**Kraemer, WJ., Noble, BJ., Culver, BW., and Clark, MJ.** "Physiologic responses to heavy-resistance exercise with very short rest periods." *International Journal of Sports Medicine,* 1987, 8:247.

**American College Of Sports Medicine.** "The recommended quantity and quality of exercise for developing and maintaining cardiorespiratory and muscular fitness in healthy adults." *Medicine and Science in Sports and Exercise,* 1990, 22:265.

**Wilmore, JH. and Costill, DL.** *Physiology of Sport and Exercise.* Human Kinetics Publishers, 1994.

**Chandler, RM., et al.** "Dietary supplements affect the anabolic hormones after weight training exercise." *Journal of Applied Physiology,* 1993, 76:839.

**Alred, HE., Perry IC., and Hardman, AE.** "The effect of a single bout of brisk walking on postprandial lipemia in normolipidemic young adults." *Metabolism,* 1994, 43:836.

**Kanter, MM.** "Free radicals, exercise, and antioxidant supplementation." *International Journal of Sports Nutrition,* 1994, 4:205.

**Moore, TJ.** *Lifespan: Who Lives Longer and Why.* Simon and Schuster, New York, 1993.

**Koffler, et al.** "Strength training accelerates gastrointestinal transit in middle-aged and older men." *Medicine and Science in Sports and Exercise.* 1992, 24:415.

**Nelson, M., et al.** "Effects of heavy resistance training on multiple risk factors for osteoporosis." *Journal of the American Medical Association.* 1994, 272:1909.

**Bevier, WC., et al.** "Relationship of body composition, muscle strength and aerobic capacity to bone density in elderly men and women." *Journal of Bone and Mineral Research.* 1989, 4:421.

**Snow Harter, C, et al.** "Muscle strength as a predictor of bone mineral density in young women." *Journal of Bone and Mineral Research.* 1990, 5:589.

**Sandvik, L., Erikssen, J. Thaulow, E., et al.** "Physical fitness as a predictor of mortality among healthy, middle-aged Norwegian men." *New England Journal of Medicine.* 1993, 328:533.

**Slattery, ML, Jacobs, DR Jr.** "Physical fitness and cardiovascular disease mortality: The US railroad study." *American Journal of Epidemiology.* 1988, 127:571.

# INDEX

chemotherapy, 90, 94
chest/bench press, 140-141, 145
China, 93, 98
chlorine, 67, 93, 113
cholesterol, 15, 89, 94, 98, 109,
    111-112, 125
choline, 80, 99-100, 114
cholycystokinin (cck), 35, 38
chromium, 77-78, 80, 89, 97, 98
cigarette, 88-90, 94, 120
circulatory system, 31
cirrhosis, 88, 93
cold, 84, 85
Colgan Institute, 68, 107-108
Colgan, Dr. Michael, 107-108
colic, 94
constipation, 15, 69, 97
Gontzea, Dr. I., 106
copper, 67, 96
cowlicks, 91
coxsackievirus, 85
cranex cranberry, 110
creatine monohydrate, 102-105
crunches, 133, 145-146
cryptococcal meningitis, 111
cycling, 107, 131, 147-150
cystic fibrosis, 93

**D**
D, L-phenylalanine, 101
dandruff, 95
DDT, 95
decosahexaenoic fatty acid (DHA),
    111-112
dehydration, 70, 110

dehydroascorbic acid, 115
deltoid, 138-141
Designer Protein - *see also protein*,
    24, 109-110
diabetes, 5, 15, 91, 94
diabetic retinopathy, 88
diarrhea, 85, 91, 95-96, 113
digitalis, 95
dilaurylthiodipropionate, 100
diuretic, 95
Down's syndrome, 94
dumbbells, 145

**E**
Eastman, 92
ECHO virus, 85
ecosopentaenoic fatty acid (EPA),
    112
elemental, 80-81, 95-96
epilepsy, 94
estrogen, 91
excipients, 116

**F**
faecium, 113
fat burning zone, 126-127, 129-
    131
fats, 15, 29, 35, 70, 89, 90, 93, 98,
    100, 107, 112
fencing, 147
fertilizers, 67, 93
fibrocystic, 99
fibrosis, 93-94
Finland, 93
flaxseed oil, 111-112

Food and Nutrition Board (FNB), 14, 80
folic acid (folate triglutamate), 78, 91
food grade, 116
football, 147-148
formaldehyde, 98
free radicals, 29-30, 67-68, 88, 92-94, 109-110, 115, 119-121, 125
fructose, 20
fruits, 3-4, 14-15, 17, 20, 31, 86, 97-98
frutooligosacchrides (FOS), 113
Fusco, Carmen, 113

**G**
gall bladder, 94
garlic, 93, 111, 113, 122
gas, 94, 102, 113, 129
gastrocnemius, 145
Georgia, 93
gingivitis, 91
gluconate, 98
glucose, 20
gluteus maximus/medius/minimus, 142
glycogen, 105, 129
goiter, 99
golf, 96, 99, 149, 150
gracilis, 143
grape seed extract, 80, 88
Greenland Eskimos, 112
gyrate atrophy 103

**H**
hamstrings, 142
hand/wrist flexors, 137, 140
handball, 147
hangover, 110
Harman, Dr. Denham, 67, 119
hayfever, 85
Healthy Choice, 4, 20, 25, 32, 33
heart disease 15, 57, 67, 92-93, 112, 117, 119
hemolysis, 105
hemorrhoids, 15
Henkel, 92
hepatitis, 86, 88, 95, 100, 165
herbicides, 67, 93, 121
hesperidian complex, 86
high blood pressure, 14, 95-97, 100
hiking, 147
Health Maintenance Programs, 76
horseback riding, 147
horseshoe pitching, 147
hypercalcemia, 97
hypothalamus, 38

**I**
iatrogenic, 122
ice skating, 147
insulin-like growth factor (IGF), 6
influenza, 85
inositol, 100
insomia, 101
insulin, 5, 6, 91, 98, 112
intermittent claudication, 92

rectus abdominus, 137
rectus femorus, 143
Reiter's syndrome, 86
Rejuvenex, 113
retina, 103
rheumatism, 81, 86, 88, 90, 93
rhomboid major & minor, 140
Ritalin, 122
Roche, 92
roller skating, 147
rollerblading, 147
rowing, 147-149
running, 87, 96, 106-107, 127,
    131, 149-150

**S**
sacrospinalis, 140
sailing, 147
sartorius, 143
schizophrenia, 89
Schwinn Airdyne, 147
scurvy, 79, 84
selenium, 80, 92-93, 95, 116
semimembranosis, 142
semitendinosus, 142
sex, 41, 89, 94
side effects, 84, 92, 99, 100, 104,
    110, 115-116
silymarin, 88
Sinemet, 90
silicon dioxide, 96
skim milk, 3-4, 17, 23, 28-29, 90,
    97
skinfold calipers, 55-57
snow skiing, 147

soccer, 149-150
sodium, 14, 17, 31, 90, 96-98, 113
softball, 147
soleus, 145
Spectrum Naturals, 112
sporogenes, 113
sports bar, 4, 24, 27, 33
Stairmaster, 147
staphylococcus, 111
stearate, 81, 96
Stone, Irwin, 86
streptococcus, 111
stroke, 14, 93, 96-97
succinate, 95
sudden infant death syndrome
    (SIDS), 78
sulfa drug, 91
sulfites, 91, 98
sulfuric acid, 67
sunscreen, 84, 91-92, 97
super sets, 145
swimming, 106, 129, 149-150

**T**
tartive dyskinesia, 99
tendinitis, 81, 87, 96
tennis, 107, 127, 148-150
teres major & minor, 140
testosterone, 94
thiodipropionic acid, 100
thyroid, 38, 99
thyroxine, 99
toxicities, 93
training zone, 126-127, 130
trapezius, 138, 140

triceps, 64, 138, 141, 145
triglyceride, 33, 89, 98, 111-112, 125
trihalomethanes, 67
TwinLab, 75-76, 102, 116
two second rule, 135, 137

**U**
ulcers, 86
urinary tract infections, 110-111
uveitis, 86

**V**
vasodilator, 89
vaginitis, 111
vastus lateralis/medialis/inter-
medius, 143
vegetables, 3-4, 14-15, 17, 20, 31-
32, 83, 86, 97-98
vegetarian, 91, 94, 105
Venezuela, 93
Vietnam war, 122
virus, 67, 79, 85, 119, 79-80, 86,
91, 100, 111
vitamin B1 (thiamin), 88, 110
vitamin B12 (cobalamin), 90-91
vitamin B2 (riboflavin), 79, 89
vitamin B3 (niacin, niacinimide),
76, 84, 89, 90, 97
vitamin B5 (calcium pantothenate), 90, 99
vitamin B6 (pyridoxine), 88, 90
vitamin C, 77-79, 80, 84-86, 89,
95, 95, 100, 110, 115,
117, 125

vitamin D-3 (cholecalciferol), 96-
97
vitamin E, 92-93
vitamin K, 96, 116
volleyball, 127, 147-148
Vitamin Research Products (VRP),
76, 96, 102, 104, 110,
113

**W**
walking, 28, 41-42, 45, 96, 126,
147, 149-150
Water Event, 69
water skiing, 147
weight training, 96, 107, 126-127,
133-134, 148-150
whey hydrolysate, 109
whole foods, 10
Wilson's disease, 94

**X-Y-Z**
zinc, 92-94, 98, 116

# TABLES AND CHARTS

**Page**

# PRODUCT INFORMATION

*The following products mentioned in the book have registered trademarks as shown below.*

| Product (TM) | Company |
|---|---|
| All-Bran and Frosted Mini-Wheats cereals | Kellogg Company |
| Fiber One, Crisp Baked Bugles, Betty Crocker Tuna Helper, and Pop Secret | General Mills, Inc. |
| Barnum's Animal Crackers, SnackWells (including picture on front cover), and Nabisco Honey Maid Grahams | Nabisco Foods, Inc. |
| Baked Tostitos and Wavy Lays | Frito Lay, Inc. |
| Cinnamon Life Cereal and Quaker Butter Popped Corn Cakes | Quaker Oats Co. |
| Healthy Choice | Con Agra Frozen Foods |
| Weight Watchers | Weight Watchers Foods |
| Lunch Bucket | The Dial Corp. |
| Star Kist Tuna | Star Kist Food Co. |
| NoSalt | RCN Products |
| Birds Eye Broccoli | Dean Foods Vegetable Co. |
| Designer Protein | Next Nutrition, Inc. |
| Coke | Coca Cola Co. |
| No Holds Bar | Natures Best |
| Power Bar | Power Food, Inc. |
| Edge Bar | Nutritional N-er-g Products |
| Pizza Hut | Pizza Hut, Inc. |
| Whataburger | Whataburger, Inc. |
| El Charrito Burrito | Don Miguel Mexican Foods Inc. |
| Delimex Beef Taquito | Delimex |
| Angela Marie's Marshmallow Munchies | Angela Marie Foods |
| Bacon Curls Microwave Pork Rinds | Curtice Burns Foods, Inc. |
| Stauffers Animal Crackers | Stauffers Foods |
| Butter Buds | Cumberland Packing Corp. |
| Mahatma Red Beans and Rice | Riviana Foods, Inc. |
| Blue Bell Light Ice Cream | Blue Bell Creameries, Inc. |
| Accu-Measure Skin Calipers | Accu-Measure, Inc. |
| Life Extension Mix | Prolongevity, Ltd. |
| Twinlab | Twin Laboratories, Inc. |
| Optizinc | Interhealth Co. |
| ChromeMate | Interhealth Co. |
| Cranex Cranberry | Physicians Natural Choice |
| Kyolic Garlic | Wanunaga of America, Ltd. |
| Nasturtium | Prima Facie, Ltd. |
| Rejuvenex | Carmen Fusco |
| N-Zime Caps | National Enzyme Co., Inc. |
| BioPro | Vitamin Research Products, Inc. |
| Stairmaster | Stairmaster Sports/Medical Products, Lp. |
| Schwinn Airdyne | Schwinn |
| LifeCycles | Life Fitness |

# NOTES

# NOTES

## ORDERING INFORMATION

To order additional copies of *Smart Eats, Smart Supplements, and Smart Exercise*, contact:

### Natural Health Solutions
P.O. Box 9407
Fort Worth, Texas 76147

or via the internet at:
http://www.spindle.net/dusty
or call local: 817-868-0220
or
1-800-484-9479, code 1825